Order this book online at www.trafford.com/07-2669
or email orders@trafford.com

Most Trafford titles are also available at major online book retailers.

Note for Librarians: A cataloguing record for this book is available from Library
and Archives Canada at www.collectionscanada.ca/amicus/index-e.html

Printed in Victoria, BC, Canada.

ISBN: 978-1-4251-5900-9

*We at Trafford believe that it is the responsibility of us all, as both individuals and corporations,
to make choices that are environmentally and socially sound. You, in turn, are supporting this
responsible conduct each time you purchase a Trafford book, or make use of our publishing services.
To find out how you are helping, please visit www.trafford.com/responsiblepublishing.html*

*Our mission is to efficiently provide the world's finest, most comprehensive book publishing
service, enabling every author to experience success. To find out how to publish your book, your
way, and have it available worldwide, visit us online at www.trafford.com/10510*

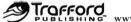 www.trafford.com

North America & international
toll-free: 1 888 232 4444 (USA & Canada)
phone: 250 383 6864 ♦ fax: 250 383 6804 ♦ email: info@trafford.com

The United Kingdom & Europe
phone: +44 (0)1865 722 113 ♦ local rate: 0845 230 9601
facsimile: +44 (0)1865 722 868 ♦ email: info.uk@trafford.com

10 9 8 7 6 5

Patient Data 101

A

`p·h·i´ Publications, Inc.

Book

Written by Kosta Tzavaras

Phi Publications, Inc.
P.O. Box 1846
Thousand Oaks, CA 91358-0846
Orders: www.phipublications.com
email: sales@phipublications.com

"This book outlines, very clearly, the options that researchers and analysts now have to measure important healthcare trends and patient behaviors. It should be required reading for anyone at any type of organization who needs an authoritative and complete education on these progressive healthcare data types and the applications for which they are best used."

- Jody Fisher, Vice President, Verispan, LLC

"Longitudinal patient and payer data can provide exceptional customer insights to help drive sales and marketing effectiveness. "Patient Data 101" is the perfect primer and reference guide to quickly get you ahead of the curve toward understanding how to select, analyze or apply this information."

- Karin Hayes, Group Director, Wolters Kluwer Health Inc.

"In an area where there's been long standing confusion around the myriad types, sources, applications and limitations of patient data sets, the insights uncovered here serve to demystify this area, putting the various data types in their appropriate place, in a way that's easy to navigate and will help not only the pragmatists but the early adopter set as well, in expanding the use of these powerful data."

- Jim Carroll, Director, IMS Health Inc.

"This book provides a useful primer for anyone interested in the current state and future development of patient data and related analytic applications, and is a thorough review of the benefits and caveats of the sources of the data for those already familiar with the subject."

- Andrew Kress, President, SDI, Inc.

Table of Contents

Preface

This book is intended for pharmaceutical and biotechnology data analysts, consultants, and data vendors with a focus in the area of patient data. It is intended to provide an introduction to the basic data concepts and uses of the data. For the novice data user, it provides the foundational knowledge to start engaging with data applications, while it expands the knowledge or clarifies ideas for the more advanced user. The book is not intended for teaching analytical, programming, or statistical methods, nor is it concerned with the implementation of healthcare software and processes.

The book focuses on two key areas: the theoretical framework of patient data and the key patient data applications. The book examines the roots of the data, its communication paths to becoming a product, the business functions that cause it to exist, the key players and stakeholders involved, and the data transformation process that results in the development of the data products. The book also directly examines the unintended applications of the data, and indirectly, its intended uses. The intended uses of the data are tied to the processes that originally generated it, and the unintended to the orchestrated efforts of manufacturers and others to influence those same processes.

Patient data may be thought of as existing in a new era when it comes to the history of data developments within the pharmaceutical industry, with the eras of sales and prescription data having preceded patient data. The development of new products, analytical capabilities, research possibilities, and generally the benefits from the gained insights have generated much excitement. Never before has the pharmaceutical industry experienced such a euphoric abundance of information, and never before have decisions been as informed as they will be the era of patient data.

Chapter 1
Patient Data

What is Patient Data?

Patient data is an organized collection of information transcribed from numerous patient encounters with healthcare providers. Every time a patient has an encounter with a healthcare provider, an electronic or manual record of that encounter is created. This is the beginning of patient data, but patient data does not exist until these records are collected and organized. In the case of a physician visit, where the episode is recorded on a patient chart, the information has a ways to go before it reaches a database. In the sole case of a pharmacy visit, however, the episode is instantly recorded in an organized data collection by the pharmacy software.

For the purpose of this book, that data collection is a commercially viable database. The central figure in the data is the anonymous patient, whose identity is concealed and is identified only by a consistent (but otherwise meaningless) patient identification number. In essence, we are talking about de-identified patient data, which is simply referred to in this book as patient data.

Patient data has in recent years received a lot of attention, and generally ranks amongst the most valuable types of data for the pharmaceutical and medical industries. Within the pharmaceutical industry, it was adopted quickly by clinical and research departments, but its commercial applications lagged until some significant database improvements in recent years. Patient data is still evolving, with small, continuous improvements being made to the existing databases in addition to new, groundbreaking ones.

Patient data was a "missing link" in the data spectrum in the sense that it focused attention on a key unit of observation that had been missing in the past from data analysis: the patient's experience. Prior to patient data, the whole experience of the patient could only be measured through inferences made from disparate pieces. Organized patient data links these experiences together in a meaningful and coherent way.

Patient data stands out because of its rich content, and in that respect, it compares to no other data type. The breadth of the data reaches from the clinical to the more financial aspects of the healthcare industry, covers all aspects of care, and can be used for scientific as well as commercial applications. The data exposes the interactions between the patient, provider, payer, and other intermediaries. It links the three important dimensions of care: diagnosis, treatment and cost.

It is because of its versatility that patient data finds use by a variety users and applications. Drug manufacturers use the data to measure clinical and economic outcomes to support their value propositions, assess and measure market potential, understand disease and treatment dynamics, optimize their marketing promotion and targeting, and to understand and deal effectively with the payer. Providers use the data to compare themselves with competitors, identify trends, assess new business opportunities by offering new products and services, and to secure their presence in the right locations. Payers use the data to stay competitive by offering clients the right benefit designs at the right price. Employers use it in benchmarks against competitors seeking to improve employee retention and productivity by offering competitive health care benefits and wellness programs. State and federal programs use it to estimate the provider costs and set reimbursement rates. Government and research organizations use it to monitor disease populations and other epidemiological data, along with treatment trends.

More importantly, the patient benefits from this through better treatments and a lower cost of care, without any threat to the patient's privacy. Both regulation and technology had a hand in ensuring that the patient identity is not compromised, even though a patient's identity is anonymously preserved in order to create the patient history that is so vital to data analysis.

The Patient Record

The origins of patient data can be traced to the patient's medical records. These records are usually scattered between a number of healthcare sites. It is rare for a single site to hold the complete collection of records over the course of a patient's lifetime. This is because patients see a number of physicians, get admitted to different hospitals, visit different pharmacies, etc., all of which are the result of relocations, employment changes, health insurance changes, aging and the onset of chronic illnesses, and other factors. As a result, the patient's medical record gets fragmented and resides within a number of general practitioner and specialist practices, hospitals, pharmacies, and other sites.

Although the primary care physician (PCP) is usually made aware of the patient's various encounters with other providers and notes the events, it is unlikely that they have enough information to accurately reconstruct the details of these encounters. A complete medical history may exist for young or healthy patients with only a few encounters. However, time erodes the completeness of that history, as these young patients age and are faced with the above scenarios. Further standard dynamics of the healthcare experience make it difficult to understand how to put any one part of the patient's activities into appropriate context. For example, a pharmacy does not record the disease the dispensed medication is used for, nor does a physician or facility know how compliant a patient is being in following their therapeutic care once the patient leaves their medical offices.

It is technological limitations that currently prevent the systematic integration of all information related to the patient's care. The use of technology for the electronic transfer of the encounter information is not widespread enough to have a significant effect on the consolidation of the patient records from other providers, either. This is because a number of healthcare sites still do not use computer technology for the exchange of information, and manual handling is impractical and prohibitively expensive. This will definitely be a much easier task in years to come, as electronic medical record (EMR) systems are more broadly adopted by the physicians' offices, clinics, and other smaller healthcare sites not currently utilizing the software.

Patient data, as a result, is not about the patient's lifetime medical history, and as we will see later, the relevance of historical data has its limitations. It is mainly about taking snapshots of patient medical history from shorter periods of time. These snapshots do not necessarily have the same start and end dates, nor do they include all types of encounters for all patients, but they are hopefully stable. What contributes to their stability is when the same healthcare services are used consistently, such as when the patient stays with the same PCP or specialist, fills the prescriptions at the same pharmacy, or stays with the same insurance plan or employer for periods of time. When enough pharmacy, physician and hospital encounters are captured, the end result is a database with a certain continuity of medical history for a number of patients; at least enough to support research projects.

Patient data studies may focus on a disease from a single aspect of care only: drug therapy, office visits or hospitalizations. In that case, only one of the patient's pharmacy, physician or hospital encounter histories is relevant. Other studies may involve a disease from both the medical and drug therapy aspects, in which case the patient's pharmacy, physician and perhaps hospital encounters specific to that disease are relevant. Finally, a study may involve multiple diseases and all types of encounters. A database may capture data history for any number of patients for each of the three types of encounters for single-focus studies. For a number of these patients, however, a cross-section of all three types of encounters must exist to support more comprehensive studies.

Data products today fall in one of two categories. The first category captures more data for each type of encounter, but has a relatively smaller cross-section of patients with a complete history. These databases are commonly referred to as "open panel" patient databases, where there is no limitation of exclusion criteria for a patient's presence in the dataset. The second category captures patients with a complete history only, but relatively fewer total patients. These databases are commonly referred to as "closed panel" patient databases, and as such, they typically restrict themselves to patients with a similar unifying criteria, such as a unique payer who has paid for all of the stops in the patient's healthcare experience. Both types of databases can support the majority of patient data applications, but also have their strengths and weaknesses with certain types of applications. There are no set limits for database size, except that a database must capture enough data representative of most or all diseases. Exception may be rear diseases and specialty databases.

Qualifying Dimensions

Realizing the limitations of the patient record, it is understood that patient databases consist of fragmented data in some way. The only reason the databases are usable is because, among the fragmentation, there exists a relatively complete treatment history for a number of patients. Sometimes the fragmentation is such that a database may contain almost random pieces of data for certain patients. The latter may not be useful in any way immediately; however, it may become relevant later if the database is enhanced with new data for the patient from new sources.

Patient studies have widely varying requirements. Depending on their composition, databases will lend themselves to some studies adequately, but will simply not support all applications. And although being able to meet the requirements of all applications is not a qualifier, random collections of patient data do not automatically make for a commercially viable database. For that to happen, a patient database must meet a number of qualifying requirements. The following are some of these requirements:

Encryption – Patient data is subject to strict HIPAA privacy regulations. When the data is used for commercial purposes, the patient identification attributes must be encrypted in a way that reasonably prevents the re-identification of the patient. Within the bounds of treatment, payment and administration interactions between provider-to-provider and provider-to-payer (where the information is used for the purpose of continuing care and reimbursement for services and certain scientific purposes), these rules do not apply. For all other purposes, the patient must be referred to by an encrypted identification number. The encrypted ID allows the patient to be identified as the same person in various transactions without revealing who the person is.

The encrypted ID is usually based on the patient name, the date of birth, gender, and geographic attributes such as the zip code, etc. Other attributes that may reveal a patient's identity, such as the cardholder identification numbers, prescription numbers, and medical record or case numbers assigned by providers or payers, are also subject to encryption in the database. The date of birth is usually not encrypted, but the day of the month is modified in order not to reveal the exact birthday, yet still preserve the year and month needed to calculate the patient's age.

Historical Perspective – The importance of historical data is that it helps establish benchmarks or reference points, as well as identify trends. Most patient data studies are non open-ended, retrospective analyses with a defined period of interest that may extend back a number of years. Some studies require that qualifying patients have historical data for specific start and end dates. Other studies require patient history for a certain length of time with varying start or end dates, or a number of months or years before or after a certain event date.

In either case, the history of the data source available becomes crucial, given the objective is to represent as much of a patient's experience as possible. A useful patient database must have enough historical perspective to deal with a range of applications. Given the pace by which the medical field is advancing in terms of diagnosing and treating diseases with the advent of new technologies, procedures and drugs, it is understood that recent history is most relevant. Over time, the patterns of care change; as newer treatments become more prevalent and older treatments are phased out, the importance of historical data more than a few years old diminishes.

Longitudinal Aspect – The mere fact that a database includes historical data does not imply that the patient is visible the entire time. For that to happen, the patient must be identifiable consistently throughout history with the same patient ID. Given the encryption requirements, that means the data would have to be reported into the database, encrypted consistently, and by the same methods for all data contributors.

Additionally, contributing data sources must supply data regularly and without interruptions for periods of time. For all patients that appear in the database, it is important that their data is depicted with a minimum of gaps. The time periods with data continuity for different patients may vary, and a patient may appear with data from January to December while another appears from March to February. However, that is not detrimental to the integrity of the database, even though it will have implications from a study design perspective. The "eligibility," or indicator that the patient's history is well represented longitudinally, should be testable using statistical controls.

Projectability
Projectability – Patient studies are hardly about the finite number of patients found in the database, but are rather concerned with a larger population. As long as the study sample is representative of that population, a study can be completed successfully either by generalizing the findings or by extrapolating them across a population. Not all databases are representative of the same population. Databases may be projectable to the total population, the total number of insured, the employed, Medicare populations, or others. Therefore, it is important to determine at the beginning of the study what the sample data represents and which databases can be projected to the population of interest.

Also, given that patient studies are disease or therapeutic area-specific, a database may include representative samples for some, but not all, diseases. Specialty databases focus only on specific therapeutic areas. A marketable and reliable database would include generalizable or projectable samples of data for the broader disease areas, or at least the area of specialization.

Patient-Centric
Patient-Centric – Most of the time, patient care involves physician visits and prescription filling; less frequently, it involves hospitalization and extended care. Mostly, it depends on the nature of illness. Studies often focus on the analysis of a specific type of care—more prominently, the pharmacy. A more comprehensive study would involve an analysis of all aspects of care, requiring cohorts of patients with available data in all settings. This requires that the database's pharmacy, medical, and hospital components not only have enough patient overlap to complete the study, but that the overlapping data periods of data coincide with the study period. A database that integrates patient history from all aspects of care, even if it is only partial, is said to be patient-centric. The patient-centric aspect of the database is a key attribute of a commercial database.

Completeness – The documentation of the patient's medical record consists of an elaborate array of data attributes. These attributes cannot be presumed to be transferable to a commercial database because they are subject to data agreements, confidentiality limitations, minimum standards, and must fall in the common domain of attributes from all data sources. In the process of transforming the source data to a commercial database, information deemed subject to the above limitations is excluded and does not make it to the final product. This affects the breadth of the database, and potentially limits its usability. Patient data must have a certain data element breadth to address numerous applications.

Updatability – For reasons we mentioned earlier, a database lacking recent updates will become obsolete once it no longer reflects the latest healthcare trends. In addition, prospective studies follow patient cohorts going forward, and depend on a constant stream of fresh data for updates. The updates may happen asynchronously as data is received. However, they must be completed by certain predefined database publishing dates. For the sake of data integrity, updates must be received from fixed reporting panels of data providers, with the exception of new reporting members. Therefore, a commercially viable database adheres to a well-defined update plan.

The frequency of updates and the data time lag are other important update aspects, and are more application-driven. Certain applications require almost real-time data and in these cases, a frequently updated database with a short time lag is preferable. Often, immediacy comes at the compromise of completeness and, consequently, the applications which require data that includes a complete set of transactions are better served by databases with a longer time lag. Therefore, the frequency of updates and time lag can be advantages or disadvantages for commercial databases.

Sources of Data

The concept of data sourcing is rather simple once one knows the process: define the required data elements, search for potential sources and execute some agreements. The data element requirements stem from client interactions, questions, and experiences with their needs. Armed with these requirements, data vendors can now search for the right data sources. The easiest way to do that is to map the path in which the data travels from point to point, and then identify potential interception points at high concentration areas. Usually, the concentration points are intermediaries that aid in the flow of data traffic or the final destination points. The mapping also helps in identifying the data stakeholders and the owners with whom to negotiate with. The figure below shows a high-level data path map.

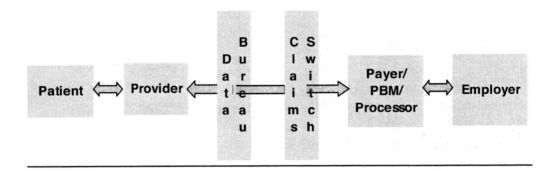

Figure 1: *Patient data flow*

The reality of patient data is that its domain is so large and its requirements so extensive that, unlike other data types, it is impossible to find one data source that meets them all. As a result, there are today a number of databases in the market with unique characteristics that fit certain applications better than others. Therefore, it is imperative that the data users understand their requirements thoroughly in order to select the appropriate data for their application. The following discussion focuses on the data sources.

The Patient - Patients initiate the first action that triggers the generation of data when they visit their care provider. The provider in turn initiates other actions with the patient, other providers, and payers, which further generates information. In the process, the patient becomes informed, and consequently this awareness becomes a source of information that when combined with input from other patients can result in a useful database.

One of the problems with the patient as a source of data is finding the right patients, who have to be identified and selected from the enormously large general population. Because of that and other reasons, no effort has been made to collect input from patients of every disease at once; rather, various initiatives address specific diseases one at a time. Patients identify themselves voluntarily through the internet, responding to mailing campaigns, magazine or media adds, or are prompted by the medical professional involved with their care. These are typically referred to as 'opt-in' programs.

The second problem with the patient as a source is often the lack of incentive for the patients to contribute their information first initially, and then routinely.

One compelling incentive for some is usually the need to receive information. Patients often resort to the internet in their search of medical information because the information they received from their professional was inadequate. This is often the case with under-diagnosed or under-treated diseases, diseases without very effective therapies, and life threatening diseases. Internet sites present patients the opportunity to receive free information, but also to contribute theirs in order to help the scientific process, which in turn has an impact on the improvement of their own condition. Patient input is usually guided to and focused towards the areas that interest data collectors. The internet boosted the significance of the patient as a source by simplifying the data collection process. Both the immediate response from the online interaction and the patient's feeling of instant gratification were the key drivers. Prior to the internet, data collection was accomplished through mail or telephone surveys. These methods are still in use today for those not adept with technology.

Some of the information patients can contribute, such as diagnosis and treatment, can be obtained from better, alternative sources, like the physician. The patient's function is as a unique source of information for measuring treatment satisfaction, preferences, symptoms, and life function information. This information is the target of patient-reported outcomes projects. Patient input is very often used in identifying outliers within the patient population, rather than validating expected outcomes. Such is the case of drug safety studies that measure adverse reactions to medications, side effects, etc.

Data collected directly from patients has certain limitations. First, the patient who lacks scientific knowledge has more subjective view of the events surrounding his diagnosis and treatment; as opposed to the professional, the patient's data may be biased towards attitude and belief. Second, the patient typically does not maintain a written record of the events, and as a result, contributes information likely to come from memory. The lack of a written record may affect the accuracy of the historical sequencing of the events. Therefore, the information patients contribute is prone to inaccuracies.

The Care Provider – This is where the vast majority of patient information is generated as a result of both the patient-provider encounter and the clinical and administrative events that take place afterwards. Clinical events include patient examination, measurement of vital signs, diagnosing, lab testing, procedures, medication administration, and prescribing. Administrative events include patient registration, validating benefit eligibility, requesting prior authorizations, and information reporting. Providers also generate financial data on the cost of care they provide to patients, pricing, and charge data, some of which they systematically communicate to payers.

Information is recorded in various ways depending on where the encounter takes place. At the physician's office, based on the current state of the technology, clinical information is recorded mostly on paper charts. The part of clinical data that will likely get transferred to an electronic form is the information that is relevant to billing. Practices are more likely to have automated billing systems, since that function is vital to the business. Less frequently, in fully automated practices, clinical information is recorded in EMR systems. At hospitals with an even greater level of automation, the events are mostly electronically recorded in real time as the orders for care are written up and the patient is moved from department to department to receive care. The patient profile, insurance information, diagnoses, medications, procedures, and tests become part of the recorded encounter and the patient's permanent record. The information is fed into the integrated billing software, where the coding staff apply the proper billing codes to generate the patient invoices and the payer claims. At the pharmacy, with the exception a few remote pharmacies that face technical challenges, the recording of data is instantaneous. This automation has primarily been driven by the urgency to complete the transaction and settle the patient charges while the patient is waiting for the medication.

This type of provider data is of the highest quality, very detailed, complete, and accurate. Up to that point, it is in its raw form and has not been manipulated in any way. The information may then be transferred electronically to business partners, such as payers or data aggregators, without much risk of reducing its accuracy. Providers also contribute information through surveys. However, surveys may be subject to different reporting rules and information transfer methods more prone to errors. Surveys are also prone to some level of subjectivity.

Providers hold pieces of a patient's medical history. Even when all of the information is transcribed in electronic form, it is difficult to communicate it electronically across providers. The standards for medical information transfers are still in development and partially in use. Much of the communication between providers is still in paper or print image form, with traditional transfer methods still in use. Currently, the incentive, obligation, necessity or the ability to coordinate the consolidation of the patient's record in one place does not exist.

The Payer – Payers, with the exception of staff model HMOs, do not provide care themselves, but simply reimburse for it. As such, they do not generate new clinical information. They do receive, however, some essential clinical information from the providers to determine the reimbursement amounts for services rendered.

Patient data is as much about clinical data as it is about financial data. The cost of healthcare is very important to many stakeholders, and the payer generates the final reimbursement figures for the insured population that quantifies it. Even though the charge figures are generated by the provider and are the basis for payer reimbursement, the burden of care is calculated based on actual payment figures. The payer also owns the plan benefit design and enrollment data outlining covered services, deductibles, co-pays, co-insurance, and covered lives. Self-insured employers own employee information such as demographics, salary, marital status, productivity data, etc. The figures for the cost of care of the uninsured are generated by the provider, who is the exclusive source of that information.

The payer comes close to solving the problem of integrating a patient's medical records. For patients with full range of medical, dental, and drug benefits, and for the period of continuous enrollment in the plan, the payer is in the unique position to capture all of their encounter data through provider-submitted reimbursement claims. The data is limited only by the partial medical information received from the providers.

Commercial third party insurers, self insured employers, Medicaid, and Medicare all fall in the payer category. Even though reference is made to the payer, often the actual touch point is not the payer, but a processor, a third party administrator, a pharmacy benefit management company, or a fiscal intermediary who represents them. Commercial payers lack access to cash paying and the non-commercial Medicaid and Medicare patient, but they do cover the managed Medicare and Medicaid patient. These are patients who sign up with a commercial insurance plan instead of the standard Medicare or Medicaid benefits. Both Medicare and Medicaid offer this choice to patients.

While a data source may serve as a holding place for data generated elsewhere, they are mostly important for the data they generate themselves. Therefore, the payer is not as important as an alternative data source for clinical data, but rather as the source of payment data. Similarly, the provider is not as important as a source of reimbursement data, but rather through the clinical data they generate.

The Software Vendor – Software vendors design, install, or support the back-end computer operations that help providers manage their business. These are typically modular systems that perform one or more functions. Pharmacy software manages inventories and purchasing, point-of-sales transactions, claims processing, disease management programs, etc. Medical practice systems handle appointment scheduling, purchasing, claims processing, manage patient care and records, etc. Hospital software, the most sophisticated and complex of all provider systems, manages all aspects of the hospital's business, including patient registration, tracking patient care and records, and claims processing.

The existence of software that tracks patient care and claims processes are the critical components of patient data collection. When available, they imply the organization of that data: a prerequisite to systematic data collection. In 2006, a survey conducted by America's Health Insurance Plans (AHIP) found that 75% of all claims were received electronically. The same survey found that in 2006, 68% of all claims were adjudicated automatically without any manual intervention. Among provider types, pharmacies have the highest level of automation, followed by hospitals, with physician practices lagging behind.

The landscape is quite different when it comes to EMR software utilization. Pharmacies, among all providers, are the least likely candidates for EMR software. The applicability of the software is rather limited to tracking side affects, allergy reactions, and for specialty pharmacies engaged in disease management programs, tracking patient outcomes. Hospitals are on the front lines, having a great degree of automation. Physician offices are now adopting the technology, but have a long way to go. Physician Practice Management companies' (PPMs) have aided the process by promoting the technology to their members. Naturally, such software offers greater advantages to physician specialties with higher degrees of complexity in the care they provide. As a result, the degree of adoption of EMR software varies by specialty. The cost of acquiring and operating the software is also a factor. The overhead associated with it is a bigger burden for solo practices and small physician groups. That is usually the reason why practices are more likely to utilize the more essential components, like claims processing, and less frequently utilize the EMR component.

Software companies are often the ones who aggregate data from the installed provider sites when they act as data bureaus on the behalf of their customers. Depending on the arrangement with their clients, they may have the right to market their data. That is often the case with the smaller providers, who cannot leverage the value of the data themselves due to its low volume, but whose data is finally of worth when pooled together with data from similar providers. Large providers like chain pharmacies, large physician practices, and hospitals are more likely to have control of their own data.

Software vendors, unlike the previous sources, do not generate new data. However, their role in the collection process is significant because they considerably reduce the tens of thousands of provider collection points, giving data vendors access to large volumes of data from a single point. Naturally, data collected from data bureaus has the same properties as the data collected from providers.

The Claims Switch (Claims Clearinghouse) – Claims switches provide the electronic platform, communication and validation software, and error checking to assure the integrity of the data transmissions. Their role is to receive, support the process of adjudication of the claim, and forward claims-related electronic transactions from providers to payers, and vice versa. Additionally, they may offer providers value-added services like data conversion and formatting for compliance with industry standards, claims editing to improve the accuracy and completeness of submitted claims for prompt adjudication and payment, and paper-to-electronic format conversions.

Their importance is characterized by the fact that they cross paths with a very significant number of patient data transactions. They can potentially accept claims from any provider and direct it to any payer, and vice versa. Because claims switches are few in number, the narrow band they form in streaming the data makes them the most efficient source for data collection.

Their business model is such that in terms of customer base, they cut across the provider and payer industries with access to a wider variety of players than any of the above data sources. Claims switches capture data only for the insured population. The broader visibility, however, comes at the expense of data completeness for some patients, as claims switches may touch data from more providers and more payers, but only obtain partial data from many of them.

Like software vendors, claims switches do not generate new clinical or financial data. However, they record details of the interactions between providers and payers that are of interest to some stakeholders. This is a rather unique feature to this source. In aggregate, the data collected from switches has the same properties as the data collected from payers; the sole exception is enrollment data, which is only available from payers.

Data Collection

From the previous discussion, it is clear that while software vendor and claims switch data mimic other sources, the patient, provider, and payer sources are unique. Data collection from these three sources has as many differences as they do similarities, which accounts for the variability among the current data products in the market. Because of the unique features of each source, a single source of data cannot entirely satisfy the spectrum of data features or information requirements. The patient perspective is only available with the patient as the source; certain clinical data can only be sourced from the provider, and benefit information only from the payer.

The unique features of these sources eventually manifest themselves in the data products, becoming the strengths and weaknesses of the databases and the basis of differentiation between them. The presence of a unique feature will make the product applicable to more applications, while the lack of it will limit the data use for some applications. These strengths and limitations are among the database design considerations of data vendors. One option data vendors often pursue is mixing data sources to compose databases with expanded features in an attempt to cover certain shortcomings. Therefore, commercial databases are not necessarily homogeneous, single source products.

Having identified the sources of the data, let's take a look at some key aspects of the data collection process. Gathering data from every collection point is not feasible for various reasons, mainly technical and economic ones. Data vendors must sort through the numerous collection points and assemble an appropriate reporting panel for the construction of their database. The following are key criteria for qualifying data collection points.

Number of collection points – In the previous discussion we identified
five potential sources for patient data collection: patient, provider, software vendor, claims switch and payer. The first obvious characteristic of these sources is the widely varying number of collection points within each one. The basic premise here is the minimization of the number of contributing sources for the maximum database size.

The number of collection points is the most important consideration of a source because it directly affects the amount of effort that goes into the collection process. There is an overhead associated with each collection point that includes the cost of data, setup, data transfer, and processing costs. Because of this, there is almost a linear relationship between number of collection points and overhead within a source, illustrated by the chart at lower-left. This differs from collecting an increased number of records from the same collection point, where the incremental overhead diminishes with each additional record – see chart at lower-right.

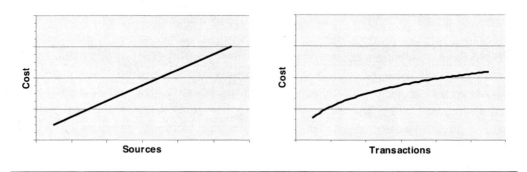

Figure 2: *Data collection cost trends*

The patient as a source of data has by far the most collection points. Each patient contributing their own data is an individual data point. These patients number from a few tens of thousands to millions, depending on the targeted disease, and that makes this the least feasible source for data collection. On the other end of the spectrum is the claims switch category, having but a few collection points. The high concentration of data through claims switches allows the buildup of large samples from but a small number of them. Software vendors representing large numbers of providers are close behind, with perhaps only a few dozen collection points. Payers, only a few hundred in number, are also efficient in data collection. National and large regional payers have millions of lives covered in their rosters, and to construct a representative sample it requires—at most—a few dozen to contribute data. Finally, the provider, with a few thousand to a few hundred thousand of them, depending on the provider type, ranks rather low in efficiency. Exceptions are the large providers with more than a few tens of sites. Vendors usually pursue the large providers directly while they resort to data aggregators for the smaller providers.

TIP: Buying groups (PPMs, GPOs) or chains often representing large numbers of provider sites offer data for sale directly as a standalone database. Data from a single collection point should be scrutinized for biases, as these groups of providers tend to share similar practices which are not necessarily representative of the general provider universe, and adversely, data analysis is never more than analysis of one specific source.

Economies of scale

Economies of scale – For the data collection process to be feasible, the data aggregators must identify any possible economies of scale to improve three aspects of the data: quality, cost and timing. Economies of scale exist in sources where large volumes of data can be found. This is simply because the cost per unit of data, the cost to apply quality checks, optimize the frequency of reporting, and optimize production timing decreases with each additional unit after one has reached critical mass. Reaching that critical mass is very important, but not a prerequisite for every data collection point. It is almost impossible to achieve economies of scale across every collection point. Instead, economies of scale should be found in a large portion of the data. Usually, where economies of scale do not exist, the cost of the data exceeds its market value.

Claims switches are ideal sources, due to the large volume of data going through the few data collection points. Similarly, software vendors and data bureaus, both having slightly more data collection points, are close behind. Payers, with just a few hundred potential data collection points, are also viable candidates. Economies of scale erode quickly when one gets to the provider category, as there are tens of thousands of data collection points. In this category, economies of scale can only be found with the larger providers representing a few thousand sites. This group includes chain pharmacies, PPM and buyer groups, hospital chains, etc.

Ultimately, the goal is to collect a representative data sample, and by limiting the data collection to one source type, that goal is jeopardized. In some cases, the solution is to blend data from more than one source. For example, you could select chain pharmacies from the provider category and supplement it with data from one or more software vendors for smaller, independent pharmacies, or blend claims switch data with payer data. The caveat with blending different source types is that there is partial data duplication, which then has to be dealt with.

Disparity of data – Data disparity is a key consideration for data aggregators because it affects the design of the database. Databases consist of defined data elements populated with a high degree of consistency. Within a specific data type, data from different collection points will have many similarities, but a few important differences. The resulting product must be based on a common domain of data fields. Unique features and elements are not necessarily usable if they are available only for part of the database. In some cases, however, and only when there is a significant sample, they can be used to model data in a larger dataset, or can even form a separate database.

Consistency between data collection points is found more often when the data is based on industry standards, as in the case of claims data, because the exchange of data is based on a common set of fields. Standardization prevents disparities across multiple data providers and helps aggregators of the data automate the flow of raw patient data into usable formats. Even then, however, the data is subject to limitations as a result of the data providers' own restrictions. Consequently, they may prevent or reduce access to certain fields. Suppliers that severely limit the breadth of the database are sometimes not selected for data reporting.

Data that is not based on a common standard may still exhibit similarities. However, it takes a bit more effort to cross-reference similar fields and integrate data into a cohesive, common format. EMR data is one such example. Because each software vendor designs their systems independently, the database definitions vary. Nevertheless, by virtue of trying to solve the same problem, these vendors often come up with predictably similar and technically compatible solutions, capturing comparable data elements.

The type of integration outlined above aims at expanding the number of records in the database. Sometimes, however, it is beneficial to link data of different types for the purpose of supplementing one source with new data features found in another. In that case, the domains of the data fields of the sources are mostly different, except for a few common fields that enable the linking. This integration does not result in incremental patient records, but rather in the expansion of fields. In fact, the end result of the combination may be a smaller database due to the limited overlap between the two. One such example, discussed later in detail, is the combination of inpatient hospital diagnoses with drug usage data with the patient ID as the common domain.

Data disparity is also important because of the level of customization required to deal with individual collection points. Among other things, it is dependent on the supplier's level of automation, the implementation of business rules and data integrity checks, and the technical capabilities of the suppliers. Some would-be data suppliers simply are not able to produce reliable data feeds.

Automation – Commercial patient databases are compiled from automated data sources. Sources that require excessive effort for the processing of their data are not good candidates for a database. The form of stored data must be such that it can be brought to a reportable state. Converting paper documents to electronic data is simply too inefficient. Computerized data sources have different levels of automation that can affect, among other things, the reporting frequency of data, publishing deadlines, and data quality. The database stability and integrity are very important attributes of marketable databases, and therefore suppliers must be able to submit the data frequently enough, meet submission timeliness, and perform all the necessary quality assurance tests. An asynchronous database based on a different set of data reporters with every update will have impermissible continuity gaps that impair its use.

Ownership – The fact that a given data source possesses a certain amount of data does not mean that it is marketable. This is because of ownership issues and the underlying agreements of the data use. This is particularly true with the intermediaries who do not generate the data, but simply process it. Typically, the intermediaries store the data on behalf of their clients and for backup and audit trail purposes, but are not automatically authorized to share it. They do engage in data marketing agreements very often, however, with their clients. Sometimes, the right to market the data goes towards credits for services offered, or in exchange for other data.

By extension, a provider may allow its software vendor to sell its data and receive credit against software upgrades and data hosting, or sometimes exchange it for benchmark reports compiled from other competitor data. Claims switches are subject to similar limitations from providers and usually require explicit agreements in order to market the data.

Ownership rights are claimed vigorously as data is recognized more and more as a very valuable asset. Patient data in particular is in high demand, and it has significant earning potential for its owners.

Value – A database meeting the previously mentioned qualifying dimensions and the data collection considerations will hold its own value. Such a database would have the breadth of both data attributes and market perspectives, the depth of a large patient sample, and would meet the necessary integrity and quality standards to be used in research applications. The value of the final database should not be confused with the value of the source data that goes into the database. The final database is a compilation of not only raw data, but also other external reference and demographic databases; because this is achieved with the substantial effort from the part of data vendors, the value of the final database product should exceed the value of the sum of its parts.

Source raw data, most of the time, does not meet many of the previous considerations to be proportionally equal in value as the final database unless it is large enough and has the breadth and depth to serve as a stand-alone database. Source data is usually small enough to be biased, lacks other perspectives, requires standardization, and is only usable when brought together with other similar data. Value is least understood by data suppliers and, therefore, it is upon the data vendor to ensure that the cost structure of the database is sound as to not price itself out of the market.

Patient Data Types

In a broader sense, a data product based on patient information should qualify as patient data regardless of the data collection method, the level of detail, or the structure of the data. A more literal and generally accepted definition, however, calls for data detail at the individual patient level longitudinally. Many of the products in the broader category predate the true patient data, and thus they are the precursors to patient data. Even though these products would not qualify for the second category, they are still useful today, though their utility might be somewhat diminished.

The reason for the variety of the patient based products is due to the varying data collection methods, the focus of the database on specific aspects of patient's care, and the source of the information. The databases tracking any type of patient metrics can be grouped into four main categories.

- Registries
- Survey
- Billing
- EMR

The patient data products with the greatest impact are relatively new. While nothing has changed with respect to a researcher's need to answer questions, patient data has allowed them to answer even more questions or answer them with more confidence. Prior to that, a researcher had to rely more on primary market research by using focus groups and chart audit studies, or rely on syndicated products, focusing on disease metrics or patient metrics.

Registries

Registries – A registry is a database of enrolled patients and their pertinent information, usually specific to a disease or a drug. Disease registries have a broader focus, and are likely to be sponsored by non-profit or commercial organizations with the purpose of advancing the sciences intended to treat the disease. Drug registries focus on one particular therapy and are sponsored by commercial organizations. Registries are formed for the purpose of collecting information from patients, with the goal of understanding the dynamics of a disease or a treatment.

The information collected may include patient demographics, medical history, treatment history and outcomes, effects of treatment on the patient's quality of life, drug side effects, and allergy reactions. Data collection typically involves an initial registration with a baseline set of information and periodic reporting thereafter. Registries have traditionally been paper-based. However, internet-based registries have been gaining a dominant position in recent years. Their ease of use and efficiencies with data entry, timing, and patient accessibility are largely to thank for that dominance.

Registries interact with the individual enrolled patients. However, their focus generally is not on the specific patient, but on collectively studying the greater patient population. Registries are usually sponsored by drug manufacturers, providers, clinical research organizations, and government organizations.

Drug manufacturers use patient registries to capture the patient perspective, particularly their experiences with the product use, product effectiveness information, attitudes towards specific treatments, and aspects related to quality of life. These are, in essence, patient-reported treatment outcomes. Registries are also used as marketing tools. Registered patients are a captive audience towards which manufacturers often direct information in the hopes of reinforcing product use. More importantly, registries play a very important role in drug safety and pharmacovigilance as part of a product's post-approval regulatory requirements. Safety and pharmacovigilance programs begin with adverse event handling, which includes the capture, coding, recording and processing of the event. Adverse events are then evaluated, written up, reviewed, and analyzed. Findings are then reported on a periodic or expedited basis.

Physicians and physician groups may sponsor or participate in disease management registries by signing up a number of patients from their case load. Data for these patients is used to form a large knowledge base about the disease and its management that participating physicians can then use to learn about new therapy trends and to compare their practices to other participants. The common goal of treating the disease provides physicians an opportunity to network with other participating physicians. Thus, registries serve as a communication platform as well. Physicians often use the knowledge gathered in these registries to publish research findings. For physicians who cannot commit to clinical trial research, disease management registries serve as an alternative way to engage in small-scale research projects.

Researchers use the pool of patients in registries to select eligible subjects for research projects. Registry data is often used by researchers to identify new trends, design clinical trials, and to develop treatment protocols to improve the delivery of care.

The major weakness of registries lies in both input validation and objectivity. Both are mitigated partially by the number of observations. An isolated observation that turns over time into a trend in the data gains validity as the number of occurrences increase. Unlike clinical trials, registries typically lack rigorous source data validation. Registries are also referred to as observational trials, but they should not be confused in any way with clinical trials. As such, registries are better suited for generating hypotheses to guide additional research, as opposed to testing hypotheses. To lend credibility to commercially-sponsored patient registries, a scientific advisory panel of leading clinicians in a particular field is often assigned to supervise the operation, the registry, or both.

Survey Databases – These databases are sourced directly from practitioner panels by using survey forms. The panels consist of recruited physicians from all relevant specialties, weighted by specialty's size. The physicians, who receive a small compensation, fill out the forms for each patient over a specified period of time or a specified number of patients so that the reported data is representative of the physician's typical case load.

Some survey databases collect data at the individual patient level. Data is then reported at an aggregate level or the patient ID is maintained to isolate data for specific patient cohorts. The collected data is either a snapshot of a patient visit or a historical perspective of a patient's experience with a disease.

Survey databases are randomized, projectable collections of data. Even though a patient's account may be recorded individually and the events captured historically, survey databases are not considered true patient datasets. The data collection method is perhaps the most significant weakness of the data. While in theory, the reported data is a copy of the physician's records, the process of reporting lacks rigorous validation.

Diagnosis and Treatment

The diagnosis and treatment databases still in use today are precursors to patient data. Syndicated databases like IMS's NDTI, Verispan's PDDA, and other custom versions fall in this category. These products sought to answers questions related to a physician's intention to treat a particular disease, what drug therapies are prescribed, where patients are diagnosed, and who pays for the treatment.

Input for the audits is collected from stratified panels of physicians from all major specialties through standard questionnaires, each of which is filled out on a regular basis. Physicians are asked to fill out the questionnaire for each patient they see on one or more pre-specified days during a reporting period. The reporting day of the week is usually varied in successive reporting periods in order for the input to be as representative as possible of the physician's case load. A separate questionnaire captures the physician's demographics.

The questionnaire is not intended to track and report data on specific patients at different reporting periods over time, but rather to project national totals from the patient sample. The aggregated data provides totals on the key following metrics:

- Diagnosis – Captures the number of visits for the primary and secondary diagnoses and other comorbid conditions. The number of diagnoses does not match one-for-one with a set of unique patients, as it includes previously diagnosed patients. Input also includes the type of facility at which the patient was seen, a disease severity indication, physician referral information, and frequency of visits.

- Drug Therapy – Captures the number of mentions of drugs prescribed, along with the dosage, form, quantity dispensed, length of therapy, number of refills, New Rx indicator, samples, and sample days. The therapies are distinguished between new and continued, with drug replacement therapies noted along with the reasons for replacement. Non-drug therapies and alternative therapies are also mentioned.

- Medical and Drug Coverage – Captures the type of insurance covering the medical services and drug prescriptions.

- Patient Demographics – Captures the patient's age, gender, race, height, weight, blood pressure, and cholesterol level.

- Physician Demographics – Captures the physician's specialty, practice type, prescription volume, and case load by insurance type.

When weighted for the specialty's size and projected nationally to the universe of physicians, the data reveals the number of patient visits by diagnosis, disease comorbidities, where patients are seen for certain diseases, and the patient referral patterns between physician specialties. The treatment data shows the percent of patients who are not treated, placed on drug therapy, and placed on alternative therapies. For drug therapies, the data shows the most common drug therapies for a disease weighted by number of mentions, typical drug dosage by indication, and length of therapy. The data also provides a view into the reimbursement landscape and how the medical services and drug therapies are likely to be paid for a particular disease.

The data becomes more intriguing when the results are broken down by patient demographics in order to provide views of disease prevalence by age group, gender and race, or the drug dosage by body mass or age group. Using the demographics of the physicians themselves, the data reveals treatment preferences by physician age group, adoption patterns for new therapies, and the specialties responsible for the diagnoses and treatment of diseases.

Diagnosis and treatment audits offer a wealth of information at a relatively low cost, and prior to patient data becoming prevalent, they were relied upon heavily. To this day, they are a good source for determining physician "intent" in the patient's experience, and they provide information on both the reason for the patient's visit and how the provider intended on treating that patient. It is noted, however, that the audit does not follow the patient beyond the scope of the interaction with the physician, which means that its ability to determine the patient's true "compliance" with the physician's intent is limited.

The audits are perceived to have significant weaknesses in the data collection process, data validation, and consistency of physician reporting. There is simply not enough incentive for the physician to commit enough resources to answer the questionnaire with the highest level of accuracy. The lack of incentive has also an affect on the vendors' ability to recruit physicians or apply high standards of recruiting. Users cite the specialty panel sizes as another weakness, with certain specialties having too few physicians surveyed. It was typical for market research analysts to commission custom studies with expanded physician panels in order to circumvent this problem.

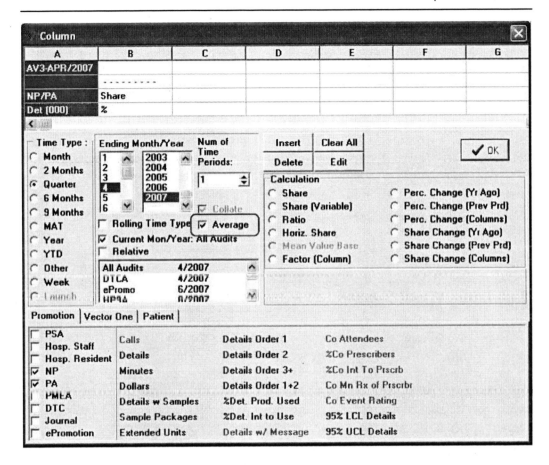

Figure 3: *Verispan's PDDA*

Even though diagnosis and treatment databases answer some of the same kind of questions as the more typical patient data, they are aggregate datasets and do not track individual patients, nor do they track data longitudinally. The more versatile patient data has taken a lot of the focus away from the diagnosis and treatment databases, although analysts are likely to consult these audits first before they undertake an expensive patient data study.

Oncology Survey Data

The oncology surveys are similar to diagnosis and treatment surveys; however, they have a narrower focus in a single therapeutic area and a more comprehensive method of data capture. Oncology, as a disease category, is much more complicated than any other disease area. The reasons lie in the multiplicity of diagnoses, indications, and the associated drug and non-drug treatments. Cancer is a chronic (but also curable) disease with the possibility of recurrence. Therefore, the patient could move in and out of the patient population several times.

The disease progresses through various stages with a chance of eventually becoming metastatic to other types of cancer, with different types of applicable treatment for each type and stage. In the process, the treatment side affects are so severe that in order to manage them, an additional battery of treatments may be necessary. Referred to as supportive therapies, these include management of anemia, neutropenia, chemotherapy-induced nausea, etc. As such, this therapeutic area requires a much more elaborate patient diagnosis and treatment tracking system. Audits in this category include IMS' Oncology Analyzer and Synovate's Tandem Cancer Audit.

These surveys use elaborate questionnaires that collect patient case data. The type of information collected covers patient and physician demographics, disease diagnosis, therapy and drug information, and supportive therapy information. The surveys target decision-making physicians in key oncology specialties, with other specialties weighted based on their level of involvement in cancer therapy. Participating physicians in the sample contribute a number of patient cases during the reporting period, based on their case load size. The sampling of physicians is varied within the reporting period so that a physician's input is randomized.

The questionnaire tries to reconstruct the patient's partial or total experience with the disease, covering initial diagnosis to subsequent stages of the disease, treatment history, and current anti-cancer and supportive therapy. Below is a synopsis of the collected data:

- Patient demographics: age, gender, weight, body mass
- Physician demographics: Specialty, practice type, practice information, affiliations, graduation, case load, clinical trial participation
- Primary cancer site and histology, metastases, comorbidities, treating specialty
- Staging at diagnosis and at subsequent relapses
- History of surgery, dates, procedures, therapeutic intent
- History of radiotherapy, start and end dates, type of radiotherapy, concurrent therapies
- History of chemotherapy, drugs, start/end dates, cycles, duration, therapeutic intent, side effects, outcomes
- Current chemotherapy, drugs, start/end dates, cycles, duration, dosage, administration, therapeutic intent, side effects, outcomes
- Supportive therapies, drugs, dosage, frequency, administration, reason for therapy, therapeutic intent

The information is recorded at the individual patient level so that specific-but-anonymous patient cases can be isolated and studied individually or in a custom cohort, yet the surveys are not longitudinal datasets. The audits provide annualized projections by cancer type. Special attention is given to the projections of patients and treatments. The same patient may have more than one treatment in the same year, and therefore in most cases, the number of patients and treatments vary significantly. The recurrence of the disease within the same year qualifies the patient as a "new" patient each time. The current disease stage, line of therapy, drug regiment and length of therapy must be analyzed thoroughly to accurately project patients and treatments.

The end product of an oncology survey database is a highly structured reporting system with an exhaustive number of outputs based on combinations of a number of detailed filtering parameters that include time periods, diagnosis, chemotherapy, drug regimens, and supportive therapy. All this may be filtered by patient or physician demographics, payer type, line of therapy, disease stage, therapeutic intent, and any other parameter collected from the input questionnaire.

Epidemiology Data

Epidemiology databases focus on another specific dimension of patient care: the number of patients in a disease category. Used for market sizing and forecasting, they track the number of diagnosed patients, the number of treated and untreated patients, and mortality and survival rates. Where applicable, the population is broken down by disease stage, line of therapy, and patient characteristics. The product of statistics, epidemiology draws from surveys, field studies, registries, national databases, patient records, and other sources to produce national and world totals. While estimating the number of diagnosed, treated, and untreated patients is possible from data available, the challenge is estimating the size of the undiagnosed patient population for a given disease.

The idea behind epidemiology in forecasting revenues for products in the pipeline is to estimate the market opportunity created by the number of treated patients. This is based on two variables: the estimated market share within the applicable lines of therapy where the product is expected to gain approval, and the product's estimated price. In reality, because of these unknown variables in the equation, forecasting is more about generating a range of possible scenarios than it is exact science. The untreated and undiagnosed populations represent, potentially, additional market opportunities for manufacturers.

Unless entirely sourced from general population surveys, epidemiological data has its roots at the patient's record. The patient's diagnosis guarantees them a place in the overall diagnosis patient count, and one of the treated or untreated counts. Epidemiology databases are byproducts of patient databases, but not true patient databases themselves. Epidemiology data addresses some of the same questions as patient data, but lacks the granularity of it. Usually, the data is aggregated at the indication level. Additionally, epidemiology databases lack the longitudinal aspect.

Billing Databases – Even though billing databases are financial instruments, they are unexpectedly able to combine both financial and clinical data. The combination of the two types of information is so powerful that it establishes these databases as the most valuable patient databases. These databases are comprehensive enough to deal with a wide range of applications, but limited enough on the clinical side to leave room for other categories of patient databases. Below is a brief description of these databases that will be discussed in detail in subsequent chapters.

- **Claims Data** - Claims databases draw from both patient financial and medical records used to generate the billing for provided care, services, and products. Pharmacy, professional, and hospital claims are compiled to form these databases.

- **Prescription Data** - Perhaps the oldest and closest type of syndicated product to patient data still in the market today is the pharmacy prescription data. Prescription data comes from the same source as the pharmacy claims data. In fact, in some instances, it is the same data as the pharmacy claims data, but aggregated and reported differently.

- **Charge Master-Level Data** - This data is patient-specific charge data itemized at the lowest level: the hospital's charge master file, a repository of detailed pricing data for all products and services offered by the hospital.

- **Hospital Discharge Data** – These databases tap into hospital claims to extract unique patient discharge information. Its primary purpose is to report the number of discharges by disease category, drug and procedure utilization, charges, and other key metrics.

EMR Data - Electronic Medical Record data is the full-fledged, patient-level medical data source. EMR data lacks the financial data elements found in claims data, but on the clinical side it goes far beyond claims. Claims data captures only enough medical detail for the payer to adjudicate the claim, and although sufficient for many data applications in most therapeutic areas, it is simply falls short for many other applications. For applications that require a more detailed account of the patient's record, EMR data is the only electronic data option and alternative to the traditional manual chart audits.

Patient Data Users

Patient data has existed in one form or another for a long time. Claims-based patient data technically begins with the early days of electronic billing, and EMR data with the beginning of practice management software system implementation. The reality, however, is that during those early days when the adoption of the software by providers was low, it would have been very difficult to compose a database and update it timely. It was not until a large enough base of providers implemented the software that data vendors found a large pool of potential data providers to recruit from

Different types of providers were slower in adopting the technology than others, with pharmacies on the forefront and physicians lagging behind. As a result, the quality of one component of the data may have been temporarily more complete than another. Also, different types of systems were adopted earlier than others, with EMR systems still lagging significantly behind claims.

These developments had an effect on the adoption of the patient data by the pharmaceutical industry. Within the manufacturer's environment, on the clinical and pharmacoeconomic sides, the value of the data was recognized immediately, and with more of a macro-focus, the early data was not significantly limited and its adoption was quicker. The smaller samples were statistically significant enough to support their respective studies. There, the health economics, outcomes, and epidemiology groups were the primary users. The main focus of such studies is the burden of illness, clinical and economic outcomes, and disease incidence and prevalence. These studies are often published in industry journals, are more thorough, and their statistical significance meticulously tested.

Meanwhile, the commercial groups with a need for broad market coverage and large data samples focused initially on prescription data. The market research and business analysis groups are the primary users of patient data for sales and marketing purposes. The focus of their studies is on treatment and utilization patterns, brand performance, and forecasting. Generally, commercial applications have a higher tolerance for error than clinical applications.

Manufacturers are not the only users of patient data. Providers, payers, and employers are also major users of the data. Their main interest is focused on industry benchmarks. Various government bodies are also interested in the data, especially those with payer responsibilities like Medicare, Medicaid, and Tricare, as well as other public health and national statistics departments. The list additionally includes independent non-profit or for-profit research organizations.

Chapter 2
Billing Databases

What is Claims Data?

Claims data is a collection of transactions initiated by providers that request reimbursement from payers for products and services provided to their covered members. A claim is initiated as a result of a patient encounter with a provider to seek care or fill a prescription. The claim typically identifies the patient and policy holder, the provider of services, the plan paying for the claim, the billed products and services, and the charges associated with them.

The provider can be any medical professional or healthcare facility, including clinics, hospitals, home healthcare companies, long term care facilities, ambulance companies, etc. The payer is any third party commercial or employer plan, Medicare, or Medicaid. Uninsured-patient and indemnity insurance transactions are settled by the patient and are the only transactions outside the standard claims process. This is a rather important fact as we will see in a later section. The patient is the person having received the services and, except for the uninsured, is named as beneficiary in the insurance policy of the policy holder. The billed products and services are a list of billable items rendered by the provider and include pharmaceutical products, supplies, lab and diagnostic tests, medical procedures, use of facilities, etc.

A claim may be submitted at the time of the service or later. Pharmacy claims are submitted during the patient visit to the pharmacy and are adjudicated with a reply back to the pharmacy before the prescription is filled. Corrections and resubmissions happen instantly during the same communication session. One exception is the few pharmacy scripts that are paid in cash by the patient and reimbursed later.

Other claims are submitted after the services are rendered, and some recurring services cannot be billed until the end of a certain period or the completion of the services. For those claims, the only interaction between the provider and the payer before or during the patient visit is when the provider verifies patient eligibility or seeks prior authorization for the services. Unlike pharmacy claims, they have a much longer processing span on average. These claims are usually more complex, require more coding and more time to review, and are more prone to errors. Corrections and resubmissions are separate events that further delay the processing, especially when manual claims are involved. Manual claims occur more frequently outside the pharmacy setting.

The Claim Process

Claims processing initially seems rather simple. It involves a recursive, two-way communication between the provider and the payer, either directly or through a claims clearinghouse. A provider submits a claim, and if the information is complete, the payer decides whether to pay the claim in whole, in part, or to reject it. The last pair of transactions in the communication, the provider's accurate claim record and the payer's response record, are the most important transactions in the whole sequence of communications. Incomplete transactions can also be important, as we will see in a later discussion.

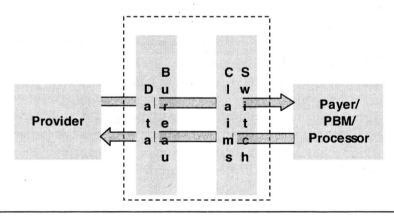

Figure 4: *Claims processing data flow*

The claims are often directed to a designated third party administrator, a processor, or a PBM designated by the Payer. Most of the claims today are submitted electronically. Generally, electronic claims are paid faster, which is enough motivation for providers to submit claims electronically. The degree of automation varies by type of provider. Without official figures, industry experts estimate that as of 2007, more than 95% of the pharmacy claims are submitted electronically, compared to approximately 90% of hospital claims and over 60% of physician office claims. Under HIPAA guidelines, providers may choose between paper and electronic claims. Under the same guidelines, payers may require providers to submit claims electronically. Medicare began requiring electronic submission in 2003, but exempted certain small providers from these requirements under certain circumstances.

When examined further, claims processing can be very complex—especially with medical claims and hospital claims, in particular. The data communicated is highly coded and requires very experienced staff to prepare and submit the claim. On the payer side, it takes sophisticated automated rule sets and qualified staff to review and settle (adjudicate) a "submitted" claim and determine if it gets "paid," "pended," or "rejected."

Paper claims must be converted to electronic form at some point in order to get paid. The void of electronic claim submission often is filled by third party intermediaries on the behalf of the provider or the payer. These companies specialize in the conversion of paper claims to electronic form. This is done by keying in the information on the form or by using automatic character recognition software.

The Standards

Healthcare provider claims fall into one of four categories: pharmacy, professional, institutional, or dental. The services provided by pharmacies, dentists, professionals, and institutions are unique enough to warrant a separate claims reporting instrument for each of them. Pharmacies, with their focus on prescription filling, require a simple, fast, and efficient reporting mechanism with minimal coding to obtain adjudication of the prescription instantly. Physicians and dentists attending the patient also require a simple reporting system to claim reimbursement for services, procedures, drugs and supplies. Institutions that deal with a complex care environment require a more sophisticated system of reporting, with an elaborate coding system to cover the myriad of services they provide and facility charges.

Reimbursement is vital to the survival of the provider's business, and that alone is enough incentive for providers to automate this process. Additionally, because manual claims processing is cumbersome and labor intensive, it is a costly operation for the provider, who can now easily justify the automation costs. For pharmacy providers, a lack of automation would mean that they would charge the patient up-front for the medication or endure the risk of unpaid claims. That in turn would shift a huge burden to payers having to process millions of manual claims from patients. For physician's practices, a lack of automation would mean a proportionally higher number of staff for each additional professional generating claims. Institutions would be faced with the same issues but on a larger scale.

For claims clearinghouses, automation was too good an opportunity to pass up. The million-plus providers on one end, in their transactions with a few hundred payers on the other end, yielded a tremendous amount of permutations of possible interfaces between providers and payers. One million providers interacting with, hypothetically, only five payers each requires five million interfaces. If on the other hand, each provider had to choose one of five claims switches (one million interfaces) to interact with their five payers, and if each claims switch maintained an interface with all five hundred payers (twenty five hundred interfaces), it would only require slightly more than a million total interfaces. Each interface associated with a certain overhead yields considerable savings that would otherwise be added to the already staggering healthcare costs. That, coupled with the error checking and quality assurance value-added services of the claims switches, further reduces costs from unnecessary re-submission of claims that both add to the overall processing costs and delay of payments.

On the receiving end, payers faced with the daunting task of processing and adjudicating the millions of claims from providers and the pressure to reimburse them on a timely fashion had no choice but to automate their processes. One of their challenges was that a number of claims were still submitted in paper form; they had to find ways to convert them to electronic form. Another challenge had to do with the millions of pieces of information that defined the claim. In order to fit every bit of that information on one side of a form, the information had to be coded extensively to avoid long strings of descriptive information. The need for coding eventually led to the development of the standards.

Payers recognized the need for standardization and made several attempts to create standards that led mainly to the development of paper forms. It was not until HIPAA's Administrative Simplification section of the law that the development and establishment of the electronic standards was accelerated, and these changes were eventually adopted by the department of Health and Human Services (HHS). In an attempt to reduce the administrative costs of healthcare, the law intended to address the standardization of electronic transmission of health information and the privacy and security issues associated with it.

The current standard for pharmacy claims is the NCPDP, Version 5.1 for telecommunications and version 1.1 for batch transactions, as specified by the

National Council for Prescription Drug Programs (NCPDP). NCPDP's Universal Claim Form (UCF) is used for submission of paper claims.

For professional claims, the paper form standard is the CMS-1500 form, and for electronic transactions, the ASC X12N 837 Professional Version. The National Uniform Claim Committee (NUCC) overseen by the American Medical Association (AMA) has the primary responsibility for maintaining these standards.

The dental claims electronic standard is the ASC X12N 837 Dental Version. The American Dental Association's (ADA) Dental Claim Form is the standard for paper claims. The responsibility for these standards maintenance belongs to the ADA and its Dental Content Committee (DeCC).

The institutional claims standard is the UB-04 paper form, previously the UB-92 form, and also known as the CMS-1450 form. The electronic standard is the ASC X12N 837 Institutional Version. The National Uniform Billing Committee (NUBC) overseen by the American Hospital Association (AHA) has the primary responsibility for maintaining these standards.

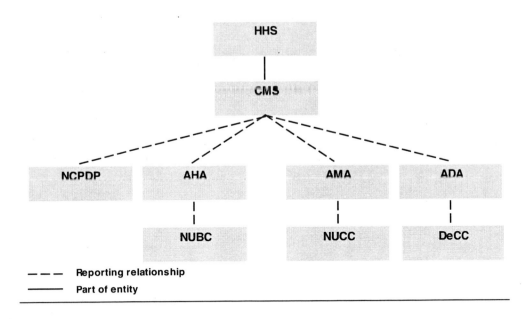

Figure 5: *Standards maintenance organizations*

While the professional, dental and institutional claims use the same electronic standard ASC X12N 837, it was determined that the pharmacy claims were unique enough and better served by the NCPDP format. Even though there are standard paper forms for filing claims, certain payers may require their own version of paper forms. The law does not mandate that claims be filed electronically, but if a provider does choose to submit claims electronically, the transmission must use the electronic standards.

In a broader context, the claim as a term could be thought of as the complete cycle of communication between the provider and payer until the transaction is settled. Literally, however, a claim is only the request for payment by the provider. The response from the payer, referred to as the remittance advice, is a separate transaction. The remittance advice transaction serves as the explanation of benefits for the claim, or it could be a payment transaction. The explanation of benefits lists payments, adjustments, patient liability, and rejections. The NCPDP standard incorporates the remittance in the same transaction as the claim but using separate segments. The ASC X12N specification uses the ASC X12N 835 transaction type for remittance.

NOTE: Claims data is usually based on both the claim and remittance transactions, and less often on the claim alone. Claims-only data is incomplete, but in some instances and where the application allows it, is a viable and (even the preferred) option because of timing reasons.

The HIPAA standards include three additional types of transactions related to the claim: the eligibility inquiry and response, prior authorization and referral, and claims status inquiry and response. However, they bear little importance to patient data because they do not feed into the data collection.

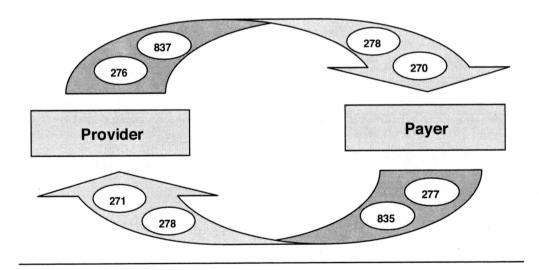

Figure 6: *ASC X12N transactions*

The Eligibility Inquiry transaction ASC X12N 270 is sent by the provider requesting clarification on the patient's benefits. The payer's reply is sent using transaction ASC X12N 271. Prior Authorization and Referral requests are sent by the provider and replied by the payer using the same transaction ASC X12N 278. Finally, inquiries on the status of the claim are sent by providers using transaction ASC X12N 276 and are replied using transaction ASC X12N 277 by the payer. Figure 6 demonstrates the ASC X12N transaction types.

In addition to file format standards, HIPAA has adopted standard medical and non-medical code sets. These are used to encode certain data elements on the claim instead of providing lengthy and cumbersome descriptions. For electronic data, un-coded data elements consume large amounts of storage space. Coding is necessary because it would be practically impossible to arrange all of the data elements on the form using full-length descriptions. The codes are translated, and full values are displayed in end-user reports as is necessary.

Medical code sets are used to describe diagnoses, medical procedures, tests, drugs and services. All other codes that do not bear clinical significance fall in the non-medical code set category. Those include state abbreviations, county and zip codes, area codes, race, ethnicity, provider type, provider area of specialization taxonomy codes, transaction type codes, reason codes, etc. Below are the key medical code sets adopted.

ICD-9-CM: The ICD-9CM (International Classification of Diseases, 9th Edition, Clinical Modifications) is a code set used to classify diagnoses and procedures, and it falls under the responsibility of the department of Health and Human Services (HHS). Volumes I and II are maintained by the National Center for Health Statistics (NCHS) and are dedicated to diseases, injuries, impairments, other health problems and their causes. Volume III is maintained by CMS and is dedicated to inpatient hospital procedures and actions for the prevention, diagnosis, treatment and management of disease, injuries, and other impairments.

HCPCS: The HCPCS (Healthcare Common Procedure Coding System) code set, also under the responsibility of HHS, has three levels of codes. Level I and II codes together are used to describe hospital outpatient or physician office procedures. The Level I procedures are also known as CPT-4 (Current Procedural Terminology, 4th Edition). CPTs are 5-digit codes and are maintained by the AMA. Level II procedures are maintained by CMS; these are 4-digit codes preceded by a character. C-codes are used for procedures qualifying for payments under the hospital outpatient prospective payment system (HOPPS). G-codes are temporary codes for professional procedures and services. J-codes are assigned to injectable and IV drug administration procedures. Q-codes are temporary codes for drugs, biologicals, procedures and services. Level III codes, also known as local codes, are designated for state specific use. With the HIPAA standardization guidelines they are now eliminated.

CDT: The Current Dental Terminology (CDT), Code on Dental Procedures and Nomenclature, Version 3 codes are maintained by the ADA and used in claims to describe dental procedures.

NDC: An NDC (National Drug Code) code is a code assigned exclusively to a pharmaceutical or biologic prescription drug. The codes are maintained and published by the HHS in collaboration with drug manufacturers. Drug manufacturers, re-packers, and re-labelers register their products with the FDA's Drug Registration and Listing System (DRLS), from which the FDA publishes the NDC directory several times a year. The NDC code is a 3-segment, 10-digit code in one of three configurations: 5-4-1, 5-3-2, or 4-4-2. The first segment is the FDA assigned registration number given to the manufacturer, re-packer or re-labeler of the product. The second and third segments are assigned by the manufacturer to identify the product and package size respectively. For standardization purposes, HIPAA has adopted a 5-4-2 format. To convert the code from the FDA format to HIPAA's 11-digit scheme, segments are padded with leading zeros as need.

Sources of Claims Data

As we saw earlier, electronic claims are initiated by the provider and sent to the claims switch so that they can be directed to the right payer or PBM. Sometimes the claim is sent directly from the provider to the payer. Any returned transactions will follow the same path back from the payer to the provider. Claims data, therefore, could be captured at any of three touch points.

Provider Claims Databases - Provider claims databases are sourced directly from chain pharmacies, group practices, clinics and hospitals or through their data aggregators. They include every claim of a provider, but only claims from participating providers. While they offer a complete perspective of these providers, they lack the perspective of the providers excluded from the sample. This is dealt with through careful design of the data sample so that it is appropriately representative of the whole universe of providers.

A patient will appear in a provider-sourced database only if at least one of their providers is captured in the database. A patient, therefore, may have all, some, or none of their medical or pharmacy history captured. For example, the database may include the patient's PCP visits but not specialist visits, or it may include pharmacy transactions but not hospital visits. Without the ability to determine what is missing, a lack of certain claims does not imply missing data, because the patient may simply not have any encounters. To include all of a patient's care, the database must capture every one of the patient's providers. Although not impossible, this may happen only for a small number of patients. A larger number of patients will have some of their pharmacy and physician visit data. The size of the cross-section of patients with some pharmacy and medical data is a very important attribute of provider claims databases.

Even though the patient's care is partly captured in the database, the continuous history of care with a provider like the pharmacy makes the data valuable. Intermediately visiting an alternative provider will cause gaps in the patient's data if the alternative provider is not a reporter. Such gaps in the database affect the results of a study. When patients switch their care to providers that are part of the sample, their data is cross-referenced, and the history continues without gaps. A patient 'drops off' the database either when they switch care to a non-reporting provider or when their reporting provider stops reporting into the database.

Provider databases are the only databases to include patients for every type of payment: cash, indemnity, third party managed care, Medicaid, and Medicare. Data observations may be generalizable or projectable to the entire patient population. Payers and plans are identified in the data by name and type. For that reason, they are very suitable for payer market share and method-of-payment analysis. Provider databases afford visibility to the prescriber and their specialties, and given their large retail data sample, they are very suitable for physician and specialty segmentation and targeting applications.

TIP: The perspective of the Medicare population aged sixty five and over is very important because it is the age group where the prevalence of certain diseases is the highest. Medicare, as a payer, maintains and markets its own claims data – see later sections.

An important consideration for provider databases is the timeliness of the data. Pharmacy claims are almost always instantly processed. Medical claims, however, have a submission delay and a lengthy processing time that together may take several months to complete. Provider databases capture and report monthly adjudicated claims from the last reporting period, with a one-month delay for data processing. Because data feeds are daily or weekly, they can report data on a weekly basis or earlier for critical applications. These are claims that were settled during the reporting month, but may originate from patient encounters from several previous reporting periods. At any given reporting period, a patient may have one or more encounters that are not yet reflected in the data. These encounters are made available as soon as their claims are settled.

Using submitted (rather than paid) claims improves the capture rate of the patient's encounters because many claims that will be settled after the reporting cut-off date are submitted before it. The biggest drawback with submitted claims is that they do not capture paid amounts—only submitted charges. However, when the data is not used for economic studies, the paid amounts are not relevant, and data based on submitted claims may perfectly suit applications that focus on clinical diagnoses and procedures. Additionally, many of submitted claims are rejected and will never make it into a database of paid claims. The fundamentals of a submitted claim do not change, however, even if the claim is rejected. An encounter for a certain diagnosis stands, whether it is paid for by the payer or not.

Provider databases are therefore quite timely, but the completeness of the patient history may be somewhat compromised during more recent time periods. To assure completeness, the data would have to be lagged several months. Even in that case, provider databases cannot guarantee the capture of the patient's complete care, and that makes these databases less useful to certain applications such as health economics and outcomes. Data timeliness is critically important to all applications that support a manufacturer's field operations.

Providers far outnumber claims switches and payers. Therefore, data collection from providers is more challenging. Data vendors look for efficiencies by contracting chains of providers, software vendors and data bureaus to reduce the data collection points as much as possible. Provider databases include IMS' LRX database, SDI's Patient View, Verispan's Vector and Wolters Kluwer's Source.

Claims Switch Databases - Data collected from claims switches includes some or all claims from a large number of providers. Claims switch databases route transactions for all types of payers (except indemnity) and capture data for almost every payer. The same patient data from different providers can be cross-referenced under the same patient ID. Cash transactions require no claim adjudication; therefore, cash-paying uninsured and indemnity insurance patients are the only patient types not captured in claims switch databases. Data observations may be generalizable or projectable to the entire insured population.

NOTE: The terms "cash-paying patient," "cash transactions," etc., refer to the uninsured and indemnity insurance patients who advance payment and are reimbursed later. Cash transactions are not transmitted to a payer. Insured patients often assume the entire cost of a transaction due to deductibles. These transactions do not qualify as "cash" in this discussion. These transactions are transmitted to the payer and are adjudicated.

Providers typically contract a primary claims switch vendor through which they submit most or all of their claims. They may also maintain a backup for black-out periods with their primary claims switch. There are instances where claims from a given provider are sent through an alternative claims switch. A claims switch will capture nearly all of the claims for providers it serves as a primary vendor for, with great continuity in the patient's recorded history. This data will have a lot of similarities with the previously discussed provider data, and patients from these providers can be expected to appear and stay visible in the database with greater predictability as long as they are cared for by the provider. For providers that the claims switch serves as a backup, the patient's history will be sparse and non-cohesive. Patients from these providers cannot be expected to appear, let alone stay visible in the database.

Because of the relatively small number of claims switches, the ratio of providers to switches is high, exposing claims switches to large numbers of providers that would otherwise be difficult to reach. Claims switch data, consequently, has great breadth of provider universe, but varying depth of patient data. Therefore, where switch claims databases may lack perhaps the complete perspective of some providers, they cover more providers than provider databases.

Some providers bypass claims switches and transmit their claims directly to payers; payers may also request direct transmissions by providers. A provider who submits claims to a number of payers is required to set up and maintain communication protocols with each individual payer, and as their contracts with payers change over time, they must establish new protocols accordingly. Claims switches inherit that task from the provider, establishing the multiple communication links between themselves and the payers and leaving the provider with a single connection point to the claims switch. The figure below demonstrates the communication connections using a claims switch.

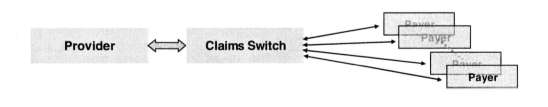

Figure 7: *Provider-switch-payer communication connections*

The high concentration of claims transaction traffic through the narrow band of switches aids the data collection process, making claims switches the most efficient among all sources to collect data. For pharmacy claims, the top three claims switches account for most of the traffic, with the largest claims switch accounting for nearly eighty percent of the traffic.

Where claims switches provide a unique perspective of the claims process is in the recording of the details through its exchanges with the payer. A submitted claim may be rejected one or more times by the payer before it is accepted because it contains errors, is missing information, fails during the transmission, etc. At other times, the claim gets withdrawn or reversed by the provider. Besides paid claims, claims switches record the rejected and reversed transactions with any applicable reason codes. Although this information is available to the providers and the payers, only the claims switch captures enough of that activity from a large number of payers to study their behavior. This behavior is critically important to the manufacturer.

One feature visibly absent from provider and claims switch-sourced patient data is plan enrollment data. There is no supplemental data to indicate when a patient signs up with a particular plan and when their coverage terminates. This information is important in data analysis when a patient's history for a particular disease is visible only for a period of time in order to determine if that is due to coverage, or the beginning or end of the therapy. With provider and claims switch databases, one must look before and after the visible period to see if the patient appears in the database with any other claims. The presence of other claims indicates that the patient was covered, but was not treated, for the particular disease.

Claims switches have to resolve data ownership issues with providers and payers, who own neither the submitted nor the responded transaction. As a result, they may be able to market a smaller portion of the larger set of transactions they record.

Payer Claims Databases – Data collected from payers includes every claim for every member patient for the enrolled period of time and for the covered services. Patients may be enrolled in one or more of a payer's medical, or pharmacy plans. Often a patient's medical coverage is with one payer but their pharmacy with another. These claims are submitted mostly by providers contracted by the payer and sometimes by out-of-network providers. The payer enters into these contracts with providers and reimburses them based on standard rates in order to manage their costs. The patient's incentive to use in-network providers comes from lower out-of-pocket expenses.

Most payers offer a variety of plans including HMO, Point of Service (POS), Preferred Provider Organization (PPO), Indemnity Fee-for-Service (FFS), Managed Medicare Part-D and Medicare + Choice, Managed Medicaid, employer plans, etc. The data lacks, however, the cash and pure Medicaid and Medicare perspectives. Payer-sourced data includes a small amount of Medicare claims for Medicare patients, with multiple coverages and Medicare as the primary payer due to a coordination of benefits. The coordination of benefits allows two or more payers to see the same claim so that they can share the payment responsibility in order of priority, depending on which one is the primary. The previous payer does not necessarily see payments by subsequent payers. Data observations in payer databases are generalizable and projectable to commercially insured population, and potentially to the entire insured population.

Patients appear in a payer database after they enroll in a plan and as soon as the first claim for a provider encounter is adjudicated. All of the patient's data is reported by the plan under the same patient ID without the need for cross-referencing. Visibility of their data is lost as soon as their coverage with the plan terminates, unless they sign up with another plan in the sample. However, patients leaving one plan for another plan in the sample appear as new patients in the database without their history being cross-referenced. Patients new to any plan in the sample are initially of little significance until they build some history with the plan; therefore, enrollment is not necessarily indicative of the strength of the database, but rather of the number of patients with a certain length of history. The history of patients no longer with the plan remains relevant for some time. Vendors will often utilize only the data for patients with both medical and pharmacy claims in their studies.

One key feature of payer-sourced data is that it comes with the patient enrollment data not available in provider and claims switch databases. Enrollment is important in determining whether the periods of inactivity in the patient's history are due to lack of patient care episodes or due to a lack of benefits. The strength of payer-provided data lies in the fact that the great majority of patients have their pharmacy, medical, and hospital claims available in the database. And in terms of provider base, payer databases cover the entire spectrum of providers, including mail order and specialty pharmacies, and institutions beyond hospitals. Unlike provider and switch databases, where the overlap of the three components relative to the size of the database is small and rather arbitrary, the overlap in payer databases is by design very significant.

Another important feature of a payer database is the patient's plan design information that comes from the participating plans. Plan design features such as formulary, benefit maximums, and other coverage options are not available in provider and claims switch databases. These databases obtain general plan design information from external databases that is not specific to the patient.

Payer databases have a time lag due to the claims adjudication process, with almost no pending transactions for the reported periods. Although pharmacy claims are more than 98% complete at the end of the reporting month, physician's office and hospital claims are only about 85% and 75% complete, respectively, three months after the reporting period. It takes approximately nine months for all claims to reach near-total completion. This apparent drawback is actually a strength in some respects. The completeness of these databases in terms of processed claims and patient history makes them uniquely suitable for a number of applications.

With payer-sourced data, the contributing payer's identity is masked in the data. Claims cannot be traced back to a payer and the participating payer list might not be known. Besides, payer coverage is limited to participating payers, and therefore, payer-level analysis is not feasible. With payer databases, analysis by plan type may be possible if the database includes a large number of plans. Payer-level analysis, such as utilization, market share analysis, and patient out-of-pocket costs, is more comprehensive with provider and claims switch databases that have full representation of the payers. Payer databases may limit the visibility to the provider by suppressing the provider IDs, unlike provider and claims switch databases. This is particularly limiting to applications requiring the physician's identity. Payers also maintain control of the encrypted patient IDs and as a result, linking of external data (i.e. consumer profiles for direct-to-patient programs) may not be possible. Lastly, payer databases may limit visibility to certain cost fields sensitive to the payer that may compromise their competitive position.

There are significantly more payers than there are claims switches, but with only a few hundred of payers in total, collecting data from payers is rather efficient. Payer databases need only to include a fraction of these payers. Payers may operate locally, regionally or nationally varying greatly in enrollment and plan options they offer. Payer databases are likely to include larger national or regional plans. The databases are composed of fixed panels of payers; therefore, they earn the title of "closed-panel" databases. Occasionally, a plan drops off or is added to the panel. Newly added plans are brought in with some history. Payer databases include IMS' PharMetrics database and Ingenix's i3.

Employer Claims Databases – This is another type of closed-panel claims database and a variation of the payer databases. The data originates from self-insured employers and the payers and PBMs hired to design and administer their medical, dental and pharmacy plans. These are the same national, regional and local payers, and PBMs that offer services of their own. These payers do not report all of their data—only the data of the employers in the panel. Where they vary from payer databases is in one area: the data sample is set around an employer panel, not around a panel of plans. An employer who terminates his or her relationship with a plan will not affect the sample, and data reporting continues with claims through the new, contracted plan. An employer's data, therefore, is not affected by plan changes.

Employer databases include claims for all enrolled active employees and their dependents, as well as retired employees who are covered by their former employers through Medicare-supplemental insurance. The data includes a few Medicare claims for this population due to the coordination of benefits between Medicare and the employer plans. Medicare in this case is the primary payer. For covered active employees or spouses qualifying for Medicare, with Medicare acting as the secondary payer, the data may not be captured. Employer plans offer a variety of plan options, including HMO, PPO, POS, and indemnity, and are projectable to the population covered by employer-sponsored insurance. Employer databases lack the cash, Medicare, and Medicaid perspectives.

NOTE: Medicare is in most cases the primary payer. Medicare is the secondary payer when the beneficiary or spouse is actively employed and covered under an employer group health plan. So that small employers are not disadvantaged, minimum company sizes (defined by the number of employees) apply for aged and disabled beneficiaries. For beneficiaries entitled to Medicare due to end-stage renal disease, Medicare is the secondary payer to a group health plan for the first thirty months of treatment.

A patient initially appears in an employer database after they are hired by a participating employer, sign up for benefits, and have their first encounter with a provider. Employees with coverage through spouses that do not enroll for the company's medical benefits are not visible in the database. They become invisible in the database as soon as either their employment is terminated, or when they terminate their benefits with the plan while still employed. Patients leaving one employer for another employer in the panel will appear to the database as new patients; their history will not be cross-referenced. New employees with little or no history under the employer plan contribute to the patient counts, but not necessarily to the usable pool of patients in studies.

For employees who sign up for the full range of benefits, employer databases capture the complete claims history for the period of enrollment, and in this sense are similar to payer databases. Patients with medical history from one plan and drug history from another are cross-referenced based on their employee ID. Employer-sourced claims databases include enrollment data and plan design information. A unique feature of an employer-sourced patient database is that it may contain productivity data such as absenteeism, short-term disability, and worker's compensation data. Productivity data linkable to medical claims allows companies to calculate the indirect costs of healthcare—a component of the total burden of illness. Employer databases also have a long lag time because, like payer databases, they include fully adjudicated claims and almost all encounters up to the end of the reporting period.

Self-insured employers outnumber payers, and vary greatly in size. The efficiencies lie in larger employers who contribute large number of patients to the database. The sample panel of employer databases is rather stable, with low turnover of employers going in and out of the plans and new employers added with some historical data. Employer databases include Medstat's patient database.

Claims Database Features - By this point, it should be clear that some features are common to all types of databases and other features are unique to certain databases. Unique features translate to strengths and advantages of any given database and make the database suitable to address specific applications. A lack of certain features would preclude a database from use with certain applications. The process of selecting a dataset should logically begin by analyzing the application requirements, determining the database type, and then settling with one of the available options. The following table summarizes data features by database type.

	Provider	Switch	Payer	Employer
Pharmacy claims data	O	O	O	O
Physician office claims data	O	O	O	O
Hospital claims data	O	O	O	O
All other Institution claims data			O	O
Fully integrated professional, hospital & pharmacy data			O	O
Some data from most providers		O	O	O
100% of a reporting provider's data	O			
Patient visible across all providers			O	O
Include all of a patient's data			O	O
Data from all methods of payment	O			
Data from most payers	O	O		
Managed care representation	O	O	O	
Medicare Part-D representation	O	O	O	
Medicare representation	O	O		
Self insured employer representation	O	O	O	O
Uninsured patient representation	O			
Projectable to total population	O			
Physician visible	O	O		
Physician specialty visible	O	O	O	O
Payer visible	O	O		
Plan type perspective	O	O	O	O
Enrollment data			O	O
Benefit design data			O	O
Employee productivity data				O
Short time lag	O	O		
Complete data for reporting period			O	O
Rejection and Reversal data		O		
True copay/coinsurance data			O	O
All Allowed and Paid data			O	O

Professional Claims

The patient's care typically begins at the physician's office, except in cases of emergency, where a patient may directly visit the ER. Therefore, the patient's diagnosis is made here first; in this, we see that professional claims hold an important piece of the patient data puzzle. Professional claims open a window of opportunity into the physician's practice, identifying patterns of care that include diagnostic and lab tests, procedures, and the usage of biologic and infusion drugs which complement pharmacy prescriptions. The physician's role is to further direct the patient to other physicians, pharmacies and institutional care as is necessary.

Consequently, physician claims are key to referral data. Furthermore, when physician claims are linked to institutional claims, the data puts hospitalization episodes in context with the patient's overall care.

The paper form standard for professional claims is the CMS-1500 developed by the Uniform Claim Task Force (UCTF) in the late 1970s. The form was most recently updated in 2005 for the implementation of the NPI identifier. The current electronic standard is the X12 837 Professional version. The first electronic standard for professional claims was the National Standard Format (NFS) developed in 1992. Both current standards are maintained today by the Uniform Claims Committee that reports to the American Medical Association.

Medicare requires electronic claims submission for non-institutional claims, unless the provider qualifies for exemption from the Administrative Simplification Compliance Act (ASCA). The role of CMS in promoting electronic claims submission is very important: because most providers treat Medicare patients, they must deal with the electronic claims submission requirements of CMS, and unless they are disadvantaged and the economic burden of implementing an electronic solution threatens their viability, they must adopt electronic claims submission.

The CMS-1500 form is organized into three sections: carrier information, patient and insured information, and physician or supplier information. The fields on the form can be logically grouped into Patient and Insured, Insurance, Patient Visit and Charges, and Provider and Physician. The data elements on the form are compatible with the electronic standard, and this discussion will focus on the CMS-1500 form for the benefit of using a visual reference.

The purpose of the discussion in this section is not to provide guidance for implementing professional claims solutions. It is intended to highlight certain data elements found in professional claims and their importance to data users with respect to patient data analysis only. Figure 8 shows a sample CMS-1500 form.

Figure 8: *CMS-1500 Form*

| 1500 |

HEALTH INSURANCE CLAIM FORM

APPROVED BY NATIONAL UNIFORM CLAIM COMMITTEE 08/05

PICA   PICA

1. MEDICARE MEDICAID TRICARE CHAMPUS CHAMPVA GROUP HEALTH PLAN FECA BLK LUNG OTHER
(Medicare #) (Medicaid #) (Sponsor's SSN) (Member ID#) (SSN or ID) (SSN) (ID)

1a. INSURED'S I.D. NUMBER   (For Program in Item 1)

2. PATIENT'S NAME (Last Name, First Name, Middle Initial)

3. PATIENT'S BIRTH DATE MM DD YY SEX M F

4. INSURED'S NAME (Last Name, First Name, Middle Initial)

5. PATIENT'S ADDRESS (No., Street)

6. PATIENT RELATIONSHIP TO INSURED Self Spouse Child Other

7. INSURED'S ADDRESS (No., Street)

CITY   STATE

8. PATIENT STATUS Single Married Other Employed Full-Time Student Part-Time Student

CITY   STATE

ZIP CODE TELEPHONE (Include Area Code) ( )

ZIP CODE TELEPHONE (Include Area Code) ( )

9. OTHER INSURED'S NAME (Last Name, First Name, Middle Initial)

10. IS PATIENT'S CONDITION RELATED TO:

11. INSURED'S POLICY GROUP OR FECA NUMBER

a. OTHER INSURED'S POLICY OR GROUP NUMBER

a. EMPLOYMENT? (Current or Previous) YES NO

a. INSURED'S DATE OF BIRTH MM DD YY SEX M F

b. OTHER INSURED'S DATE OF BIRTH MM DD YY SEX M F

b. AUTO ACCIDENT? PLACE (State) YES NO

b. EMPLOYER'S NAME OR SCHOOL NAME

c. EMPLOYER'S NAME OR SCHOOL NAME

c. OTHER ACCIDENT? YES NO

c. INSURANCE PLAN NAME OR PROGRAM NAME

d. INSURANCE PLAN NAME OR PROGRAM NAME

10d. RESERVED FOR LOCAL USE

d. IS THERE ANOTHER HEALTH BENEFIT PLAN? YES NO *If yes*, return to and complete item 9 a-d.

READ BACK OF FORM BEFORE COMPLETING & SIGNING THIS FORM.
12. PATIENT'S OR AUTHORIZED PERSON'S SIGNATURE I authorize the release of any medical or other information necessary to process this claim. I also request payment of government benefits either to myself or to the party who accepts assignment below.

SIGNED _____ DATE _____

13. INSURED'S OR AUTHORIZED PERSON'S SIGNATURE I authorize payment of medical benefits to the undersigned physician or supplier for services described below.

SIGNED _____

14. DATE OF CURRENT: MM DD YY ILLNESS (First symptom) OR INJURY (Accident) OR PREGNANCY(LMP)

15. IF PATIENT HAS HAD SAME OR SIMILAR ILLNESS. GIVE FIRST DATE MM DD YY

16. DATES PATIENT UNABLE TO WORK IN CURRENT OCCUPATION MM DD YY FROM TO MM DD YY

17. NAME OF REFERRING PROVIDER OR OTHER SOURCE

17a.
17b. NPI

18. HOSPITALIZATION DATES RELATED TO CURRENT SERVICES MM DD YY FROM TO MM DD YY

19. RESERVED FOR LOCAL USE

20. OUTSIDE LAB? YES NO $ CHARGES

21. DIAGNOSIS OR NATURE OF ILLNESS OR INJURY (Relate Items 1, 2, 3 or 4 to Item 24E by Line)

1. _____
2. _____
3. _____
4. _____

22. MEDICAID RESUBMISSION CODE ORIGINAL REF. NO.

23. PRIOR AUTHORIZATION NUMBER

24. A. DATE(S) OF SERVICE
From To
MM DD YY MM DD YY

	B. PLACE OF SERVICE	C. EMG	D. PROCEDURES, SERVICES, OR SUPPLIES (Explain Unusual Circumstances) CPT/HCPCS MODIFIER	E. DIAGNOSIS POINTER	F. $ CHARGES	G. DAYS OR UNITS	H. EPSDT Family Plan	I. ID. QUAL.	J. RENDERING PROVIDER ID. #
1								NPI	
2								NPI	
3								NPI	
4								NPI	
5								NPI	
6								NPI	

25. FEDERAL TAX I.D. NUMBER SSN EIN

26. PATIENT'S ACCOUNT NO.

27. ACCEPT ASSIGNMENT? (For govt. claims, see back) YES NO

28. TOTAL CHARGE $

29. AMOUNT PAID $

30. BALANCE DUE $

31. SIGNATURE OF PHYSICIAN OR SUPPLIER INCLUDING DEGREES OR CREDENTIALS (I certify that the statements on the reverse apply to this bill and are made a part thereof.)

SIGNED _____ DATE _____

32. SERVICE FACILITY LOCATION INFORMATION

a. b.

33. BILLING PROVIDER INFO & PH # ( )

a. b.

NUCC Instruction Manual available at: www.nucc.org

APPROVED OMB-0938-0999 FORM CMS-1500 (08-05)

CARRIER

PATIENT AND INSURED INFORMATION

PHYSICIAN OR SUPPLIER INFORMATION

Patient & Insured Information – The patient information is subject to HIPAA privacy rules and is used in the encryption algorithm of provider and claims switch sourced databases. The Patient's Name, Patient's Zip Code and Patient's Birth Date may used to generate the encrypted Patient ID. By using the common patient parameters for pharmacy, institutional and professional claims, data vendors are able to come up with consistent encrypted IDs to cross reference the claims for a patient, even though they come from different sources. The Patient's Birth Year and Sex are not encrypted. The form allows for up to two insurance policies to be specified when the patient is covered by more than one policy. These policies may be held by different individuals. The Insured's or policy holder's information does not bare any significance in data analysis with professional claims.

Patient's Name
Patient's Address
Patient's City
Patient's State
Patient's Zip Code
Patient's Telephone
Patient's Birth Date
Patient's Sex
Patient Relationship to Insured
Patient Status Marital/Employment-Student
Insured's ID Number
Insured's Name
Insured's Address, City, State, Zip Code
Insured's Telephone
Insured's Date of Birth
Insured's Sex
Other Insured's Name
Other Insured's Date of Birth
Other Insured's Sex

Insurance Information – The Insurance information section identifies the primary and secondary payer and plan of the claim. The identification of the payer is essential to payer-level analysis. The plans in professional claims are different than the plans identified in pharmacy claims. Professional claims fall under the patient's medical benefit and are reimbursed by a medical plan, as opposed to the pharmacy claims that fall under the drug benefit and are reimbursed by a pharmacy plan. With the exception of the reimbursement of office procedures involving the administration of drugs, the medical benefit does not impede the patient's access to prescription medication and, therefore, it does not impact the manufacturer nearly as much as the drug benefit plan does.

As a result, the manufacturer does not put much emphasis on the payer or plan analysis components of medical claims, and the rigor of analysis of the payer and plan seen in the pharmacy claims is missing with respect to professional claims. This analysis is more important to the payers and providers, purely for competitive purposes. Closed panel databases do not allow visibility to the payer but they provide a type of plan indicator. Payers in closed panel databases are identified with an encrypted ID.

Carrier Name
Carrier Address
Carrier City, State, Zip Code
Type of health insurance coverage
Patient's Condition Related to
Insured's Policy Group or FECA Number
Insurance Plan Name or Program Name
Employer's Name or School Name
Other Health Benefit Plan
Other Insured's Policy or Group Number
Other Insurance Plan Name or Program Name
Other Employer's Name or School Name

The "Carrier" is the entity that receives and processes the claim. This may be the payer itself or a third party administrator. The "Insured's Policy Group Number" and "Insurance Plan Name" fields indicate the primary insurance policy with "Other Insured's Policy Number" and "Other Insurance Plan Name" the secondary. The "Insured's Policy Group Number" is the policy or group number of a commercial plan. When the claim involves an accident, it is an automobile insurance policy number. For work related injuries, it is a worker's comp. policy or a FECA (Federal Employees Compensation ACT) number. The "Insurance Plan Name" sometimes may be populated with the payer ID instead.

Most data vendors do not cross-reference or standardize the plan information to a payer/plan database. Without the cross referencing, the ability to analyze the payer may be limited. That ability is further limited when it comes to the plan. Aggregations of payer data would be based on free text fields with some chance of matching the same payer, but with some variation in the values as well. Worse yet, the "Group Number" identifying the plan is usually an alphanumeric code, the meaning of which is obscure without some kind of decoding.

Patient Visit and Charges – The patient visit information on the form is without a doubt the most important section on the CMS-1500 form. Prescription claims filed by the pharmacy providers correspond (most of the time) to a professional claim. Information from the diagnosis fields provides the indication for the pharmacy-dispensed medication that was missing from the script. Additionally, information coded in the procedure field accounts for the remaining drug use not captured in pharmacy, hospital and other institutional claims. Physicians do not ordinarily medicate patients in the office, except for drugs requiring administration under the supervision of professional nursing staff. Physicians purchase and stock the drugs for which they are compensated by the payer; in addition, they receive an administration fee. The remaining procedure information describes the non-drug therapies and helps complete the treatment path data for the patient.

Date of Current Illness/Injury/Pregnancy	
First Date of Same or Similar Illness	
Dates Patient Unable to Work From/To	
Hospitalization Dates Related to Current Services From/To	
Medicaid Resubmission Code/Original Ref. No.	
Prior Authorization Number	
Diagnosis or Nature of Illness or Other Source	Occurs up to 4 times
Date(s) of Service From/To	
Place of Service	
EMG	
CPT/HCPCS	
CPT/HCPCS Modifier	
Diagnosis Pointer	
Charges	
Days or Units	
EPSDT Family Plan	
Outside Lab/Charges	
Total Charge	
Amount Paid	
Balance Due	

The "Date of Current Illness/Injury/Pregnancy" is the first date of the current episode of the disease, and if the disease has occurred in the past, the "First Date of Same or Similar Illness" field indicates such.

The "Dates Patient Unable to Work From/To" and "Hospitalization Dates Related to Current Services From/To" fields provide some measure of another aspect of the disease burden, which is the indirect economic impact of illness to employers. However, the information is rather incomplete without some employee profile information, such as hourly wage rates; here, employer-sourced data is likely to provide a more accurate measure.

The "Prior Authorization Number" may be required by certain payers for certain treatments. However, when multiple procedures are listed, it cannot be determined which procedures require prior authorization.

The form allows for up to four "Diagnosis Codes" in no particular order; they do not indicate the primary diagnosis of the patient. For any prescriptions the patient fills subsequent to the physician visit, the diagnosis codes can be used to match the drug's closest indication to the disease described by the diagnosis code. The matching of drugs to diagnosis codes is done empirically or by using references such as the ICD9-CM diagnosis reference list and the Uniform System of Classification (USC) drug reference list. The data will sometimes reveal drug usage for non-indicated diseases.

The diagnosis codes are also useful in measuring disease incidence and prevalence in epidemiology. The presence of a diagnosis in the patient's record qualifies the patient to be counted in the prevalence bucket. A newly diagnosed patient within a specified time period might qualify for both the incidence and prevalence buckets. Incidence and prevalence are more meaningful when projected to the total population.

The "Date(s) of Service From/To" field primarily indicates a single date, and is the actual date the services were provided. In a few cases, and while identical services are provided on consecutive dates, the provider may group services for those dates by providing the "From/To" dates and the "Days or Units" field to indicate the count of services. The "Date(s) of Service From/To" is very important in sequencing the patient care events when pharmacy and hospital claims are all linked together.

The "Place of Service" is a code that describes the facility type where the physician rendered his or her services. That might be the physician's office, a hospital, a clinic, a rehabilitation center, nursing home, hospice, etc. This field can be useful in determining where certain procedures are most often performed. While the office is the most frequent place of physician-to-patient encounters, physicians may provide their services in any of the aforementioned facilities.

The "EMG" field indicates whether an emergency was associated with the visit. Due to inconsistent use of the field, its reliability in data analysis may be limited.

The "CPT/HCPCS" and corresponding "Modifier" fields describe the procedures performed and drugs administered during the visit. While the above diagnoses provide a measure of disease incidence and prevalence, the procedures in the CMS-1500 (taken together with the procedures of the UB-04 form and the drug usage from the pharmacy claims) provide a measure of the treated vs. untreated patients and their respective treatment modes. Each procedure may be accompanied by up to four "Procedure Modifier Codes," the purpose of which is to provide clarity in regards to the procedure. The procedures are mapped to diagnosis codes on the form using the "Diagnosis Pointer" to indicate the reason they were performed.

The "Total Charge" is the sum of the "Charges" field. The "Amount Paid" indicates any amounts paid by the patient or other payer for covered services, and the "Balance Due" is the amount due to the provider from the payer billed. The information on the form is pre-adjudication information, and therefore, the amounts are subject to payer adjustments. As such (and consistent with other claim types), while they provide an approximate measure of healthcare costs, the most accurate figures come from the remittance advice data that comes back from the payer.

Provider and Physician – This section identifies the provider and the referring and rendering physicians. Provider and physician information is useful in targeting and segmentation. A physician's influence in a therapeutic area can be measured by the number of relevant diagnoses they make, the number of pharmacy prescriptions they write, and the procedures and drug administrations they perform. While the physician's influence in the retail drug market is easily measured using pharmacy claims, the ability to determine which physicians are responsible for the drug administrations within the office setting has been generally an unmet need for manufacturers. Professional claims now provide a viable solution, subject only to a potential suboptimal coverage of the physician universe.

At this time, professional claims samples are not as significant as pharmacy data samples. As a result, they provide only partial physician coverage. For professional claims sourced through providers or their software vendors, the physician visibility is as poor as the number of providers that report into the database. The relative importance of these providers is measurable, because the data includes all of their claims. For switch sourced claims the visibility may be wider. However, the ability to capture the relative importance of the physician in professional claims may be poor because of the partial capture of a physician's claims.

The referring patterns of healthcare are also very important to manufacturers, not so much at the physician level, but rather at the specialty level. It is important for manufacturers to identify the common diagnosing specialties and their initial or subsequent treatment actions. The physician may choose, depending on their specialty and the disease severity, to treat the patient or refer them to a specialist.

Name of Referring Provider or Other Source
Referring Provider ID Qualifier
Referring Provider ID
Referring Provider NPI Number
Rendering Provider ID Qualifier
Rendering Provider ID Number
Rendering Provider NPI Number
Federal Tax ID Number
Service Facility Location Information
Billing Provider Info & PH#
SSN/EIN
Accept Assignment

The "Referring Provider" can be identified by cross referencing their provider ID to one of the industry standard databases, depending on the type of ID provided. Similarly, the specialty may be derived through cross referencing. A common source for specialty codes is the AMA. The AMA has defined approximately two hundred physician specialties. An alternative method to determine the specialty of physicians is by the type of procedures they perform. This method classifies physicians in fewer, more general specialty categories, but cannot place physicians in more refined specialty classifications.

The "Rendering Physician" is a provider other than the billing physician who has rendered all or part of the services related to the claim on the behalf of the billing provider. The rendering physician's NPI and other ID is provided only next to the applicable procedures listed on the claim. If no rendering physician is associated with a procedure, the billing provider is assumed to have rendered the services.

When a physician orders services from a third party and bills for the services on their behalf, the "Outside Lab" field indicates such. The amount charged is indicated in the "Outside Lab Charges" field and it is payable to the entity indicated in the "Service Facility Location Information."

The "Billing Provider" is a physician or a business entity; they may be a sole proprietorship or a group practice. The billing provider's NPI number and a secondary ID assigned by the payer can be used to identify the billing entity. The Billing Provider's Tax ID is unique to the entity receiving payment. When not encrypted, this field can be used to cross-reference physicians to group-practice commercial databases.

Pharmacy Claims

The pharmacy typically is the patient's second stop after the visit to a physician. Naturally, pharmacy claims are the most important type of claims for the manufacturer because they capture drug utilization. Yet, because pharmacy claims data cannot definitively establish the relevance of drug utilization to diseases (due to its lack of diagnosis data and the existence of competing non-drug therapies), pharmacy claims data by itself provides suboptimal levels of analysis. Pharmacy claims data is important first because it quantifies drug utilization, and second because it associates usage to the physician and the payer, the influence of which the manufacturer tries to manage.

The standard for submitting pharmacy claims was developed by the National Council for Prescription Drug Programs. It is applicable to retail, mail order, specialty and long term care pharmacies, or any other pharmacies for which the drug is not reimbursed under the medical claim. The NCPDP[1] is an ANSI accredited organization, designated by HIPAA as the standard setting entity for pharmacy claims. It was formed in 1977 to study pharmacy standardization by a Senate Ad Hoc Committee. In 1978, it developed a Universal Claim Form (UCF) for billing pharmacy claims.

Pharmacies began implementing computer systems in the 1970s. Initially, they submitted computer generated paper claims on forms designed by the insurance companies, with each company using their proprietary form. In 1987, PCS was the first to introduce electronic claims, with other payers and PBMs following suit. PCS used a proprietary file format and the telephone line to receive claims directly from pharmacies. By using computer technology, pharmacies gained some processing efficiency, but they had to use separate connection hardware for each PBM. The redundancy of the multiple forms evolved to a redundancy of connection hardware and file formats for the multiple insurance companies.

The first electronic standard, NCPDP version 1.0, was developed in 1988 and allowed software vendors to focus on a single file format. Furthermore, the introduction of claims switching technologies by ENVOY/WebMD and NDC Health eliminated the need to maintain multiple connection hardware. Claims were now submitted real-time and responded in real-time. NCPDP released subsequent

---

[1]   **"Materials Reproduced With the Consent of ©National Council for Prescription Drug Programs, Inc. 2007 NCPDP"**

versions 3.2 in 1992, version 3.3 in 1996, version 4.0 in 1997, and version 5.0 in 1999. The current telecommunication standard is NCPDP version 5.1 for on-line interactive claims processing and NCPDP version 1.1 for batch transactions. The batch standard was designed for bundling a number of electronic claims together, but still uses NCPDP version 5.1 as the detail record.

The standard is designed to support pharmacy claims for drugs, professional pharmacy services, and supplies. It also supports a few other types of transactions: eligibility verification, prior authorization, control substance reporting, and information reporting. For the purpose of patient data, the transactions of interest are the claims, and therefore, we will focus our discussion on these transactions. The term "transmission" in NCPDP is equivalent to a claim, and contains up to four line items (transactions) for reimbursement. A transaction is equivalent to a prescription for a drug or a charge for a service. Therefore, a payer may be reimbursing for a maximum of four prescriptions per claim.

The standard is a comprehensive collection of data elements that are used to communicate the details of the claim. Because it is designed to account for all possible scenarios, it includes fields that are not frequently populated. From the patient data standpoint, not all fields are useful for data analysis. Depending on contracts made, a vendor database may include all or part of the NCPDP data field set. The complete NCPDP set of fields covers the spectrum of possibilities with regards to pharmacy claims.

Figure 9: *Universal Claim Form (UCF) © NCPDP*

CARDHOLDER I.D. ______ GROUP I.D. ______

CARDHOLDER NAME ______ PLAN NAME ______

PATIENT NAME ______ OTHER COVERAGE CODE (1) ______ PERSON CODE (2) ______

PATIENT DATE OF BIRTH ___ MM ___ DD ___ CCYY ___ PATIENT (3) GENDER CODE ______ PATIENT (4) RELATIONSHIP CODE ______

PHARMACY NAME ______

ADDRESS ______ SERVICE PROVIDER I.D. ______ / QUAL (5) ______

CITY ______ PHONE NO. (   ) ______

STATE & ZIP CODE ______ FAX NO. (   ) ______

FOR OFFICE USE ONLY

WORKERS COMP. INFORMATION
EMPLOYER NAME ______
ADDRESS ______
CITY ______ **STATE** ______ **ZIP CODE** ______
CARRIER I.D. (6) ______ **EMPLOYER PHONE NO.** ______
DATE OF INJURY ___ **MM** ___ **DD** ___ **CCYY** ___ **CLAIM (7) REFERENCE I.D.** ______

I have hereby read the Certification Statement on the reverse side. I hereby certify to and accept the terms thereof. I also certify that I have received 1 or 2 (please circle number) prescription(s) listed below.

PATIENT / AUTHORIZED REPRESENTATIVE

ATTENTION RECIPIENT PLEASE READ CERTIFICATION STATEMENT ON REVERSE SIDE

TYPE OR PRINT ALL INFORMATION NEATLY AND COMPLETELY IN APPROPRIATE SPACES

(PERF)

1

PRESCRIPTION / SERV. REF. #	QUAL. (8)	DATE WRITTEN MM DD CCYY	DATE OF SERVICE MM DD CCYY	FILL#	QTY DISPENSED (9)	DAYS SUPPLY

PRODUCT / SERVICE I.D.	QUAL. (10)	DAW CODE	PRIOR AUTH # SUBMITTED	PA TYPE (11)	PRESCRIBER I.D.	QUAL. (12)

DUR/PPS CODES (13)	BASIS COST (14)	PROVIDER I.D.	QUAL. (15)	DIAGNOSIS CODE	QUAL. (16)
A B C					

OTHER PAYER DATE MM DD CCYY	OTHER PAYER I.D.	QUAL. (17)	OTHER PAYER REJECT CODES	USUAL & CUST. CHARGE

1	
	INGREDIENT COST SUBMITTED
	DISPENSING FEE SUBMITTED
	INCENTIVE AMOUNT SUBMITTED
	OTHER AMOUNT SUBMITTED
	SALES TAX SUBMITTED
	GROSS AMOUNT DUE SUBMITTED
	PATIENT PAID AMOUNT
	OTHER PAYER AMOUNT PAID
	NET AMOUNT DUE

2

PRESCRIPTION / SERV. REF. #	QUAL. (8)	DATE WRITTEN MM DD CCYY	DATE OF SERVICE MM DD CCYY	FILL#	QTY DISPENSED (9)	DAYS SUPPLY

PRODUCT / SERVICE I.D.	QUAL. (10)	DAW CODE	PRIOR AUTH # SUBMITTED	PA TYPE (11)	PRESCRIBER I.D.	QUAL. (12)

DUR/PPS CODES (13)	BASIS COST (14)	PROVIDER I.D.	QUAL. (15)	DIAGNOSIS CODE	QUAL. (16)
A B C					

OTHER PAYER DATE MM DD CCYY	OTHER PAYER I.D.	QUAL. (17)	OTHER PAYER REJECT CODES	USUAL & CUST. CHARGE

2	
	INGREDIENT COST SUBMITTED
	DISPENSING FEE SUBMITTED
	INCENTIVE AMOUNT SUBMITTED
	OTHER AMOUNT SUBMITTED
	SALES TAX SUBMITTED
	GROSS AMOUNT DUE SUBMITTED
	PATIENT PAID AMOUNT
	OTHER PAYER AMOUNT PAID
	NET AMOUNT DUE

NCPDP UNIVERSAL CLAIM FORM (UCF)

SCREENS: BOX 10%, TEXT 11%.

The following section discusses the various segments in a pharmacy claim and their fields. The discussion is not intended as a guide to implementing pharmacy claims systems, but as a guide to patient data for pharmaceutical manufacturers. The purpose of it is to identify the key data elements and put their importance in context with patient data analysis.

To better organize the data around the functions performed, the file format logically groups related fields together into segments. Segments and data fields may be mandatory or optional depending on the function performed. Optional fields may not be populated, and optional segments may not be submitted. The standard outlines the mandatory and optional segments and fields for each function. Pharmacy claims data is based directly on input from these fields and segments.

Transmission Header	Occurs once per claim
Patient Segment	"
Insurance Segment	"
Prescriber Segment	Occurs up to four times per claim
Pharmacy Segment	"
COB/Other Payment Segment	"
Worker's Compensation Segment	"
Claim Segment	"
Drug Utilization Segment	"
Coupon Segment	"
Compound Segment	"
Pricing Segment	"
Prior Authorization Segment	"
Clinical Segment	"

When a number of claims are sent together in batch mode, a Batch Header segment is used to mark the beginning of the batch and identifies the sender and batch number, creation date, and time. The "Sender ID" identifies the provider. A Batch Trailer Segment is also used to mark the end of the batch and provides the number of records in the batch. The batch number in the Batch Header segment must match the batch number of the Trailer Header segment. The batch number is also used to match payer responses to submitted claims. The "Transaction Type" field has a value of "T" when the pharmacy is submitting the batch and "R" for responses to the claims by the payer. A value of "E" indicates that the whole batch was rejected due to errors.

Transmission Header Section - This segment appears once per individual claim or once for each claim in a batch. It identifies the routing destination, the type of transmission, the pharmacy or provider, and the date of service.

BIN Number
Version Release Number
Transaction Code
Processor Control Number
Transaction Count
Service Provider ID Qualifier
Service Provider ID
Date of Service
Software Vendor/Certification ID

The "BIN Number" or "Bank Identification Number" identifies the card issuer and is used as a network destination for routing electronic transactions to claims processors. Using the BIN number, the provider or claims switch can guide a transaction to the right payer, PBM, or processor. The BIN Number is a six-digit number issued by ANSI. BIN numbers are found worldwide on credit, debit, charge, and other cards to identify the network they belong to. In the United States they are also found in NCPDP pharmacy claims.

The 'Processor Control Number' (PCN), when required by the payer, is assigned by the claim processor to identify a payer or a payer's plan. In some cases, the same PCN may be used for multiple payers. The "BIN Number" and the "Processor Control Number" are coded data elements used by data vendors to identify the processor and the payer responsible for the reimbursement in the claims transactions. The decoding of the payer and processor is critical to payer-level data analysis.

The "Transaction Code" identifies the type of transmission. Pharmacy billing transactions have a Transaction Code of "B1." When a claim is already adjudicated but the patient fails to pick up the prescription, the pharmacy reverses the transaction to void the payment request. Reversals have a transaction code of "B2." When a change to a claim occurs, the claim must be re-billed. Re-bills have transaction codes of "B3" and imply a reversal of the previous billing, which must take place before the new billing is processed.

NOTE: A reversal cancels an approved claim transaction, and a re-bill is a duplicate transaction. Reversed and duplicate re-billed claims are not included in paid claims data.

Patient Segment - The patient segment identifies the person who received the healthcare services. This is a person named in the insurance policy, but does not necessarily have to be the policy holder. This is a key segment in the claim, and even though the patient information is not available in claims databases as shown below, its availability (even in encrypted form) ensures the longitudinality of the claims databases. Below is a list of the key fields in this segment:

Patient ID Qualifier
Patient ID
Date of Birth
Patient Gender Code
Patient First Name
Patient Last Name
Patient Street Address
Patient City Address
Patient State/Province Address
Patient Zip/Postal Zone
Patient Phone Number
Patient Location
Employer ID
Smoker/Non Smoker Code
Pregnancy Indicator

Due to HIPAA privacy guidelines, the fields in this segment may be encrypted or not provided. The patient's first and last name, date of birth, and zip code are used to produce the encrypted patient ID, and are typically present in the data submission (but encrypted). Other encrypted fields may include the "Cardholder ID" and the "Prescription/Service Number" found in other segments. The year of birth and gender do not need to be encrypted based on the HIPAA guidelines.

Vendors use combinations of encrypted fields to create a unique patient ID. Encryption is done in such a way that the ID cannot be reversed-engineered to reveal the identity of the patient. The encryption of the patient's information in subsequent claims, using the same algorithm, would yield the same patient encrypted ID, which then allows all of the patient's claims to be linked. The linking of patient claims by different pharmacies and other providers is only possible if the same encryption engine is used at every data collection site.

Insurance Segment - This segment identifies the cardholder and the insurance plan that reimburses the claim. Payer and plan-level data analysis are two of the

71

key applications of pharmacy claims data. Payer actions related to drug benefit designs (such as formulary product preferences / restrictions and patient burden) directly affect drug manufacturers. Patient out-of-pocket expense, prior authorization, claim rejection, and claim reversal analysis at the plan level enables the manufacturer to focus on plans where they might be disadvantaged when compared to other manufacturers. Medical plans impact the manufacturer significantly less.

Cardholder ID
Cardholder First Name
Cardholder Last Name
Home Plan
Plan ID
Eligibility Clarification Code
Facility ID
Group ID
Person Code
Patient Relationship Code

The "Cardholder ID" is one of the encrypted fields in the claims databases. Along with other patient encrypted fields, it may be used to assign the patient a unique ID. The "Person Code" identifies each covered person, and the "Patient Relationship Code" indicates the patient's relationship to the cardholder.

The "Plan ID" is a processor assigned code that indicates benefit or coverage criteria. It usually distinguishes between HMOs, PPOs, IPA plans, etc. The "Group ID" is a number assigned to the cardholder group or employer group. The Plan and Group IDs are critical to identifying the insurance plan by name. These are not "intelligent" IDs, and data vendors must decode them through various methods. Payers use the BIN, PCN, Group ID, Plan ID, and Cardholder ID fields to organize their business. Collectively, these fields provide the information needed to identify the payer and plan from the data.

Pharmacy Segment - This segment identifies the pharmacist dispensing the medication or the person responsible for the provision of the services billed. The provider is identified by one of many IDs. However, with the implementation of the National Provider Identifier (NPI) number, each provider will be identified by a unique NPI in all claims data. The identity of the pharmacy is usually restricted in data applications and the information in this segment has limited use. Pharmacy-level data may be used in benchmarking studies and pharmacy ranking applications.

Prescriber Segment - This segment identifies the prescriber. It is also intended to identify the patient's primary care provider when it is not the same as the prescriber, although such information is often not populated in the claim.

This is a key segment, as the prescriber information found here is used in targeting and segmentation applications that use patient data. Traditionally done using prescription data, the additional parameters found in claims data now provide significant advantages for their use in these applications over prescription data. Pharmacy claims databases and prescription databases are essentially different cuts from the same pharmacy data, although prescription databases use larger samples.

The prescriber information is also useful in identifying referral patterns in the progression of the disease. One may, for example, identify the role of the general practitioner and specialist during the early stages of a disease and note how that changes in later stages. An initial prescription by a PCP and a subsequent prescription by a specialist for the same patient and same disease would indicate referral with initial treatment. A diagnosis by a PCP from physician claims without a prescription and a prescription by a specialist would indicate a referral without initial treatment. Some patient databases restrict the use of the physician name but allow for specialty-level analysis.

Note: Physician specialty is not one of the NCPDP fields, but it is introduced by the data vendors by matching the prescriber to industry standard physician databases.

| Prescriber ID Qualifier |
| Prescriber ID |
| Prescriber Location Code |
| Prescriber Last Name |
| Prescriber Phone Number |
| Primary Care Provider ID Qualifier |
| Primary Care Provider ID |
| Primary Care Provider Location Code |

COB/Other Payment Segment - This coordination of payment (COB) segment is applicable when the patient has supplemental coverage and the claim is paid by more than one payer. Its purpose is to inform the other payers of partial payments made on the claim, or the reasons for any claim rejections. The claim is submitted to the primary payer first, and then forwarded to any additional carriers to reimburse for any unpaid amounts by the previous payers.

COB/Other Payments Count	(max 3)
Other Payer Coverage Type	Occurs up to 3 times
Other Payer ID Qualifier	Occurs up to 3 times
Other Payer ID	Occurs up to 3 times
Other Payer Date	Occurs up to 3 times
Other Payer Amount Paid Count	**(max 9)**
Other Payer Amount Paid Qualifier	Occurs up to 9 times
Other Payer Amount Paid	Occurs up to 9 times
Other Payer Reject Count	(max 5)
Other Payer Reject Code	**Occurs up to 5 times**

The file format allows for up to three additional payers in the claim record. For each payer, the provider may specify up to nine amounts paid to include coupons, or up to five rejection codes. Providers must submit the claim to the next payer after a response is received from the previous payer, which in essence generates multiple claims. Data vendors are able to remove duplicate claims because they all reference the same prescription number. Only the last in the chain of transactions captures the total reimbursed amounts and lists all of the payers. The primary carrier would be designated as "Other Payer (1)."

Worker's Compensation Segment - This segment is applicable when the claim is work-related. The segment lists the date of injury, the employer name, address, telephone number and contact, and the "Carrier Code" assigned in the Worker's Compensation Program. This is not a required segment of the claim and the information is rather underutilized in patient data analysis.

Claim Segment - This is the most important segment in the claim, as it lists the drugs dispensed and services rendered by the pharmacy. For the manufacturer, pharmacy patient data is first about drug utilization and treatment patterns, with physician / payer influences and the economic impact of drug therapies encompassing secondary concerns.

Rx/Service Reference# Qualifier	(01=Rx Billing, 02=Service Billing)
Rx/Service Reference Number	
Product/Service ID Qualifier	

Product/Service ID	
Associated Rx/Service Reference#	
Associated Rx/Service Date	
Procedure Modifier Code Count	(Max 4)
Procedure Modifier Code	Occurs up to 4 times
Quantity Dispensed	
Fill Number	
Days Supply	
Compound Code	
Dispense As Written (DAW)/Product Selection Code	
Date Prescription Written	
Number of Refills Authorized	
Prescription Origin Code	
Submission Clarification Code	
Quantity Prescribed	
Other Coverage Code	
Unit Dose Indicator	
Originally Prescribed Product/Service ID Qualifier	
Originally Prescribed Product/Service Code	
Originally Prescribed Quantity	
Alternate ID	
Scheduled Prescription ID Number	
Unit of Measure	
Level of Service	
Prior Authorization Type Code	
Prior Authorization Number Submitted	
Intermediary Authorization Type ID	
Intermediary Authorization ID	
Dispensing Status	
Quantity Intended To Be Dispensed	
Days Supply Intended To Be Dispensed	

A pharmacy claim is most often for a prescription, and in very few cases, for a service. The "Prescription/Service Reference Number Qualifier" indicates the type of billing for the claim. A value of "1" indicates a prescription, and a value of "2" indicates a service. Services offered by pharmacies may include measuring the patient's vital signs, recording a patient's medical history, counseling and education and referrals to specialists, etc. Service claims presently have very limited data application.

The "Prescription Reference Number" is unique to an original prescription and each associated refill. Payer responses to claims are matched back to the original transaction using this number. For dispensing, the "Product ID" is typically the NDC number of the drug. The "Product ID" is a very important data element of pharmacy claims. Data vendors cross-reference the NDC numbers to national databases to identify the product, its form, and its strength. The "Fill Number" indicates an original fill when the value is zero or the re-fill number, if re-fills are allowed as indicated in the "Number of Refills Authorized" field. For service billings, the "Service ID" values provide the CPT-4, CPT-5 or HCPCS codes associated with the procedures performed when the "Service ID Qualifier" has a value of "07", "08", or "09." The "Procedure Modifier Codes" provide clarifying information on HCPCS procedures.

The "Quantity Dispensed" and "Days Supply" are very essential pieces of information from which the average daily dosing information is calculated. The calculation of the average daily dose is necessary because there is no specific dosing information captured on the claim. The "Unit of Measure" clarifies how the quantity is measured, be it in milliliters, grams, etc. For partial prescription fills with "Dispensing Status" marked as "P" (Partial) or "C" (Complete), the "Quantity Dispensed" and "Days Supply" reflect the actual dispensed amount and days with the "Quantity Intended to be Dispensed" and "Days Supply Intended to be Dispensed" containing the written values on the prescription. The "Associated Rx/Service Reference Number" and "Associated Rx/Service Date" in a subsequent complete fill reference the initial partial fill transaction. Partial fills are usually due to inventory shortages.

Prescriptions are not always filled as prescribed. The "Originally Prescribed Product Code" and "Originally Prescribed Quantity" fields are intended for that purpose. Therapeutic and generic substitutions directly affect drug manufacturers and are indicative of the payer's control. The information in these fields can be used to analyze substitutions due to pharmacist intervention before a claim is submitted. For substitutions after a claim is rejected, analyzing sequences of submitted, rejected, and approved transactions from claims switch-sourced databases, when taken together with the rejection codes, provides a more comprehensive view.

The presence of a "Prior Authorization Number" in the claim indicates a possible barrier set by the plan for the manufacturer's drug. Prior authorizations are common with new drugs and in cases where payers try to prevent or control the use of a drug, typically in favor of other drugs in the formulary. Analysis of prior authorization data, together with patient out-of-pocket expense and claim rejections, are used to quantify a plan's influence.

DUR/PPS Segment - This segment is intended for the pharmacist to clarify the reasons for an intervention in the drug therapy due to drug use review (DUR). Reasons may include conflicting drugs in therapy, adverse reactions, drug allergies, dosage conflicts, a pregnancy indicator, etc. For Professional Pharmacy Services (PPS), the segment is used by the pharmacist to list the services provided such as patient assessment, consultation or education, medication review, selection, or administration, etc. This is not a required segment of the claim, and the information is rather underutilized in patient data analysis.

Coupon Segment - This segment is used only when a coupon is submitted by the patient. Coupons are usually issued by manufacturers to reduce the patient's out-of-pocket expense by providing a price discount on a cash prescription, reducing the co-pay, or by offering free products. Coupons intended to reduce the co-pay are submitted to the coupon processor after the claim has been adjudicated by the primary payer. For free product or cash prescriptions, the coupon is submitted directly to the coupon processor.

The coupon processor appears to the pharmacy as a payer with its own BIN, PCN, and Group ID numbers, which are usually imprinted on the coupon. The coupon processor claim is the last claim when a primary payer is involved. Therefore, coupon processing may require multiple transactions for processing. Unlike claims involving secondary insurance carriers, however, the coordination of benefits segment may not be submitted to coupon processors, in which case the full reimbursement information may not be on the coupon claim.

Coupons are found in the pages of newspapers and magazines or mailed to patients by manufacturers. They are also given out by physicians in lieu of samples. Coupons require a prescription from a physician. From the patient data standpoint, a coupon for free product is much preferred over a physician dispensed drug sample because it leaves a record of the filled script. The script then becomes part of the patient's medical history due to the claim submission to the processor. A drug sample left at the physician's office has very little chance of being recorded electronically.

Coupon Type
Coupon Number
Coupon Value Amount

The "Coupon Type" indicates if the coupon is good for a price discount, free product, or other reduction of cost. The "Coupon Number" is the serial number assigned to the coupon. The "Coupon Value Amount" can be a specific dollar amount, a percent price reduction, or may not have a specific value when good for free product. In the last case, the "Usual and Customary Charge" of the pharmacy is the amount reimbursed to the pharmacy.

Compound Segment - This segment is applicable only for compounded products. Each ingredient in the formulation is listed separately along with its cost. The compound's total cost is the sum of the cost of all of its ingredients and it is reported in the claim in the "Ingredient Cost Submitted" of the Pricing Segment. The compounded product is a drug with its own form, unit of measure and route of administration. The "Compound Dosage Form Description Code," "Compound Dispensing Unit Form Indicator," and "Compound Route of Administration" capture that information. The resulting product, for example, may be a 50ML syrup that is administered orally. Information from this segment is not frequently used in data analysis.

Pricing Segment - This segment lists the pharmacy charges for the products and services rendered, allocated to the appropriate categories and responsible parties. However, because the pricing is set by the payer, the submitted charges may not match the paid amounts that are outlined in the payer's response transaction. The payer may override any amount, including ingredient and dispensing fees, based on contracted pricing. Exceptions to this are the cash-paid prescriptions, for which this segment is the only available source. From the data analysis standpoint, the paid charges are more important than the submitted charges. Depending on the source of data, some databases may include submitted, paid, or both types of charges.

Ingredient Cost Submitted	
Dispensing Fee Submitted	
Professional Service Fee Submitted	
Patient Paid Amount Submitted	
Incentive Amount Submitted	
Other Amount Claimed Submitted Count	(max 3)
Other Amount Claimed Submitted Qualifier	Occurs up to 3 times
Other Amount Claimed Submitted	Occurs up to 3 times
Flat Sales Tax Amount Submitted	
Percentage Sales Tax Amount Submitted	
Percentage Sales Tax Rate Submitted	
Percentage Sales Tax Basis Submitted	

Usual and Customary Charge
Gross Amount Due
Basis of Cost Determination

All of the above fields in this segment are intended for pharmacy use. However, because of payer contracts and agreed pricing, the pharmacy may not populate these fields. The "Ingredient Cost Submitted" is the most basic charge of the dispensed script. The "Basis of Cost Determination" field clarifies how the ingredient cost was calculated, i.e. AWP, acquisition, direct, etc. In addition to the ingredient cost, there may be dispensing fees, and taxes (flat or percentage). Shipping and administrative charges are captured in the "Other Amount Claimed Submitted" field. Incentives paid to pharmacies for dispensing specific contracted drugs or services are submitted in the "Incentive Amount Submitted" field. All of the above amounts are aggregated in the "Gross Amount Due" field. The formula to aggregate the gross amount due is as follows:

Gross Amount Due = Ingredient Cost Submitted + Dispensing Fee submitted + Incentive Amount Submitted + Other Amount Claimed Submitted + Flat Sales Tax Amount Submitted + Percentage Sales Tax Amount Submitted

The "Usual and Customary Charge" is the amount cash-paying customers are charged excluding tax or other potential charges. It is provided in a claim only as a reference to the claimed amount. The "Patient Paid Amount Submitted" is the patient's out-of-pocket cost for the prescription. That amount, and any other amounts paid by any other payers captured in the "Other Payer Amount Paid" in the COB segment, are deducted from the "Gross Amount Due" to determine the "Net Amount Due" to the pharmacy. The formula below shows the calculation of the net amount due:

Net Amount Due = Gross Amount Due – Patient Paid Amount Submitted – Other Payer Amount Paid

Prior Authorization Segment - This segment is used by the pharmacy to obtain prior authorization from the payer to dispense a drug not in the formulary that would most certainly be rejected if submitted in the claim. It is submitted before the therapy is initiated to assure that the pharmacy will be reimbursed for the products or services.

Prior authorizations are typically valid for a period of time or a certain number of refills. The exceptions are granted by the payer and based on medical necessity due to interactions or adverse reactions of formulary drugs, combination therapy with drugs already on formulary, etc. Once a "Prior Authorization Number-Assigned" is given by the payer, the number must be submitted in the "Prior Authorization Number Submitted" field in the claim segment, otherwise the claim may be rejected.

Although pharmacy requests for prior authorizations are supported by the NCPDP standard, a prior authorization is often obtained by the physician, who in turn provides the authorization number to the pharmacy so that they may submit it in the claim. Prior authorization is critically important in the analysis of a payer's formulary control. The consistent presence of a prior authorization number in claims for a product indicates a barrier to product use that is imposed by the payer. The analysis, however, does not make use of this segment, but uses the "Prior Authorization Number Submitted" field in the claim segment.

Clinical Segment - This segment is used in conjunction with claims for professional pharmacy services. It lists up to five diagnosis codes, along with date, time, and the patient's clinical values (as measured by the pharmacist during an examination). These services are not frequently performed. In fact, some pharmacies simply do not offer them. Clinical information is almost never submitted by the pharmacy in a drug dispensing claim, and that is a key difference between professional and institutional claims.

NOTE: The new and developing trend of the retail clinic may give a whole new meaning to the clinical segment. Retail clinics are store-based clinics staffed mostly by nurse practitioners to diagnose and treat minor conditions. Pharmacies are well positioned to adapt to this model, and initial indication is that they will engage in it. If payers allow pharmacies to claim reimbursement using the NCPDP standard for these services, this segment will be much more frequently used. In fact, it will be a very important source of diagnosis data. However, payers may require submission of a professional claim instead, in which there will be no change in the way this segment is utilized.

A submitted claim generates a response back from the payer. Similar to submitted claims, batch submissions are answered in batches bundled between the Batch Header and Batch Trailer Segments. Responses are also organized in segments. Certain segments in the response apply to the claim while others are specific to a prescription or service in the claim. The Response Header Segment captures the acceptance or rejection status of the whole claim. Claims with errors and non-qualifying claims are rejected with the appropriate messages sent back to the provider. The Response Status Segment is used to communicate the approval or rejection status of a prescription in the claim. For approved claims, the Response Pricing Segment includes the reimbursement information. Data from the response segments is very important in two ways. First, it includes the actual reimbursed amounts. Second, the rejection codes carry significant importance in commercial applications. The information allows drug manufacturers to analyze rejected claims and focus on coverage issues with payers that do not favor the use of their products. Pharmacy patient data is based on a combination of submitted and response transaction segments. Below are the segments in a claim response.

Response Header Segment	Occurs once per claim
Response Message Segment	"
Response Insurance Segment	"
Response Status Segment	Occurs up to 4 times per claim
Response Claim Segment	"
Response Pricing Segment	"
Response DUR/PPS Segment	"
Response Prior Authorization Segment	"

Response Header Segment - This segment indicates if the transmission of a claim was successful. The segment includes some transaction identification information in order to reference the response to the submitted claim. Most of the fields in this section correspond to the submitted Transmission Header Segment, with the same values used to pair the response to the request.

Version/Release Number
Transaction Code
Transaction Count
Header Response Status
Service Provider ID Qualifier
Service Provider ID
Date of Service

The "Header Response Status" indicates if the transmission of the claim is Accepted (A) or Rejected (R). Claims that are rejected due to transmission errors must be resubmitted. Errors in the Transaction Header Segment, Patient Segment or Insurance Segment of a submitted claim trigger the rejection of the whole claim. This type of rejection automatically triggers the rejection of all transactions in the claim.

Response Status Segment - This segment indicates if a specific transaction in a claim is Paid (P), Rejected (R), or Captured (C) for later processing. This segment is critical for filling the prescription. A rejected drug prescription may be approved with a subsequent claim and proof of medical necessity, or it may be substituted with an approved drug. Alternatively, the patient would have to pay cash.

Segment Identification	
Transaction Response Status	
Authorization Number	
Reject Count	(max 5)
Reject Code	Occurs up to five times
Reject Field Occurrence Indicator	Occurs up to five times
Approved Message Code Count	(max 5)
Approved Message Code	Occurs up to five times
Additional Message Information	
Help Desk Phone Number Qualifier	
Help Desk Phone Number	

The "Transaction Response Status" indicates if a prescription within a claim is accepted or rejected. An error in any segment other than the Transaction Header Segment, Patient Segment, or Insurance Segment of the submitted claim triggers a prescription-level rejection. An accepted claim may have any combination of captured, paid, or rejected transactions. For example, the payer may pay for a drug in the claim but reject another for payment. The rejection of a single transaction in the claim does not result in the rejection of the whole claim.

For a rejected transaction, there can be up to five "Reject Codes." The "Reject Count" indicates the number of codes. For a paid transaction, there can be up to five "Approved Message Codes," as indicated in the "Approved Message Codes Count." For rejected transactions, the "Approved Message" fields are blank, and vice versa. The payer uses the "Approved Message" fields to suggest the pharmacist's future actions, such as generic and formulary drug utilization. The "Additional Message Information" is a free-form text message specific to the transaction.

The rejection codes are of the most importance in this segment. There are more than two hundred rejection codes defined in the V5.1 standard. Most of the codes are field edits for missing or invalid values or codes related to processing errors. As such, the importance of them is rather insignificant from the patient data standpoint because they do not have a business impact, other than requiring input correction and resubmission of the transaction or claim. The significant rejection code categories are related to patient coverage, benefit design, and prior authorization issues. All three categories affect drug manufacturers and may represent a missed opportunity. Manufactures then have an opportunity to address these issues by examining formulary issues with the payers and educational programs for physicians and pharmacies.

Response Claim Segment - The response claim segment is limited to the prescription identification number for pairing claims with responses. It is also used by the payer to reply back to the pharmacy with the preferred products for the substitution of a rejected product.

Prescription/Service Reference Number Qualifier	
Prescription/Service Reference Number	
Preferred Product Count	
Preferred Product ID Qualifier	Occurs up to six times
Preferred Product ID	Occurs up to six times
Preferred Product Incentive	Occurs up to six times
Preferred Product Co-pay Incentive	Occurs up to six times
Preferred Product Description	Occurs up to six times

The "Prescription/Service Reference Number" is identical to the one in the submitted claim. The "Preferred Product ID" is usually the NDC code or other ID as is indicated in the "Preferred Product ID Qualifier." A higher "Preferred Product Incentive" for the pharmacy and a lower "Preferred Product Co-pay Incentive" for the patient are motivating factors to switch products.

Response Pricing Segment - This is another key segment of the claim, as it highlights the economic considerations of healthcare and is the basis for pharmacoeconomic studies. In this segment, the payer itemizes the reimbursed amounts for the products and services rendered by the pharmacy, and allocates the costs to the appropriate categories and responsible parties.

Segment Identification
Patient Pay Amount
Ingredient Cost Paid
Dispensing Fee Paid
Tax Exempt Indicator
Flat Sales Tax Amount Paid

Percentage Sales Tax Amount Paid
Percentage Sales Tax Basis Paid
Incentive Amount Paid
Professional Service Fee Paid
Other Amount Paid Count
Other Amount Paid Qualifier
Other Amount Paid
Other Payer Amount Recognized
Total Amount Paid
Basis of Reimbursement Determination
Amount Attributed to Sales Tax
Accumulated Deductible Amount
Remaining Benefit Amount
Amount Applied to Periodic Deductible
Amount of Co-pay/Co-insurance
Amount Attributed to Product Selection
Amount Exceeding Periodic Benefit Maximum
Basis of Calculation-Dispensing Fee
Basis of Calculation-Co-pay
Basis of Calculation-Flat Sales Tax
Basis of Calculation-Percentage Sales Tax

Many of the fields in this segment correspond to the submitted pricing segment. In this segment, the payer advises the pharmacy of the patient's out-of-pocket expense in the "Patient Paid Amount" field, and of the total reimbursed amount in the "Total Amount Paid" field. The net amount due to the pharmacy is calculated by first adding up the ingredient, dispensing, incentive, sales tax, shipping, and administrative fees, and then subtracting the patient's responsibility amount and any other amounts paid by other payers when there are multiple insurance plans, including coupons.

Total Amount Paid = Ingredient Cost Paid + Dispensing Fee Paid + Incentive Amount Paid + Other Amount Claimed Paid + Flat Sales Tax Amount Paid + Percentage Sales Tax Amount Paid – Patient Pay Amount – Other Payer Amount Recognized

The "Patient Pay Amount" comprises any and all of the following: "Amount of Co-pay/Co-insurance," "Amounts Attributed to Periodic Deductible," "Amount Attributed to Sales Tax," "Amount Attributed to Product Selection" and Amount Attributed to Periodic Benefit Maximum." The "Patient Pay Amount" is always available from the payer. However, the components of it are sometimes not populated. Therefore, the ability to analyze the patient out-of-pocket costs by component will vary in difficulty by the availability of these key data elements.

"Amounts Attributed to Periodic Deductible" are usually applicable at the beginning of the covered period and until the patient has paid one hundred percent of the drug costs for up to a set amount. The co-pay and co-insurance are set by the plan and are applicable for the remaining benefit period after the deductible amount has been met and before the benefit maximums have been met. Co-pays are fixed amounts within defined tiers, regardless of the cost of the drug dispensed. For example, in the generic tier, the co-pay may be five dollars; in the branded tier, it may be ten dollars; it may be twenty dollars for biologics. Co-insurance is expressed as a percent of the patient's responsibility of the overall cost. A patient, for example, may pay ten percent of the prescription cost while the payer pays the remaining amount. The benefit design requires a co-pay or co-insurance, but not both. Amounts due to product selection may result from the patient's choice of a premium drug, instead of a generic or a drug in the formulary. The patient is usually asked to pay the difference between an equivalent covered drug and the selected drug. These costs are also applicable during the entire covered period and do not count towards the deductible. The patient is also responsible for any amounts in excess of their maximum allowed amount by their plan design for the covered period. These costs go towards the later part of the covered period, as the patient exhausts his or her benefits. "Amounts Attributed to Sales Tax" are infrequent, though they are applicable during the entire covered period.

The payer may or may not populate the "Accumulated Deductible Amount" and "Remaining Benefit Amounts" fields. The "Basis of Calculation" of the dispensing, co-pay, and sales tax fields is provided for clarification.

Institutional Claims

In the pharmacy claims discussion section, we saw how drug utilization, its associated economics, and the physician and payer's influences were the key points of interest. By contrast, the drug utilization data garnered through institutional claims is rather limited to outpatient; the physician visibility, although important, can be somewhat difficult to gauge; the payer influence is less important and differs significantly from pharmacy claims. The main focus in the analysis of institutional data lies in disease dynamics and the economics thereof. This mostly non-drug data is still very relevant to the drug manufacturer because of the way it impacts drug utilization. Because institutional care is very expensive, manufacturers often base their value propositions on the premise that proper drug treatments prevent hospitalization and reduce health care costs.

The diagnosis of the patient that was absent in the pharmacy data is available here in abundance, and the procedure data provides visibility to the other types of treatments beyond drug use, especially when used in conjunction with professional and pharmacy claims to construct the complete treatment profile of the patient. The payer is not under much scrutiny here due to the fact that reimbursement schemes for drugs are different. However, the economics are very important from a macro level.

Institutional claims are filed either through paper forms or electronically. The paper claim form is used by providers exempted from CMS' mandatory electronic claim submission or third party payer requirements. The first paper form standard for institutional claims was the UB-82, introduced in 1982 by the National Billing Committee, which was commissioned by the American Hospital Association in 1975. Prior to that, there had been several initiatives that failed to produce an acceptable standard. UB-82 was subsequently replaced by form UB-92 ten years later. The form was revised again and approved in 2005, and form UB-04 replaced UB-92 in March of 2007.

The ASC X12N institutional electronic standard has been in use since 2003. The UB-04 data elements map to corresponding fields in the ASC X12N format and both standards are designed to meet the same requirements. Both standards use the same codes as well. Since the two standards are equivalent, for the purpose of this book our discussion will focus on the UB-04 standard for the benefit of using a visual reference. Figure 10 demonstrates the UB-04 form.

Figure 10: *UB-82 Form*

1		2		3a PAT. CNTL #			4 TYPE OF BILL
				b. MED. REC. #			
				5 FED. TAX NO.	6 STATEMENT COVERS PERIOD FROM THROUGH		7

8 PATIENT NAME	a		9 PATIENT ADDRESS	a			
b			b		c	d	e

10 BIRTHDATE	11 SEX	12 DATE	ADMISSION 13 HR	14 TYPE	15 SRC	16 DHR	17 STAT	CONDITION CODES 18 19 20 21 22 23 24 25 26 27 28	29 ACDT STATE	30

31 OCCURRENCE CODE DATE	32 OCCURRENCE CODE DATE	33 OCCURRENCE CODE DATE	34 OCCURRENCE CODE DATE	35 OCCURRENCE CODE	OCCURRENCE SPAN FROM THROUGH	36 CODE	OCCURRENCE SPAN FROM THROUGH	37
a								a
b								b

38			39 CODE	VALUE CODES AMOUNT	40 CODE	VALUE CODES AMOUNT	41 CODE	VALUE CODES AMOUNT
			a					
			b					
			c					
			d					

42 REV. CD.	43 DESCRIPTION	44 HCPCS / RATE / HIPPS CODE	45 SERV. DATE	46 SERV. UNITS	47 TOTAL CHARGES	48 NON-COVERED CHARGES	49
1							1
2							2
3							3
4							4
5							5
6							6
7							7
8							8
9							9
10							10
11							11
12							12
13							13
14							14
15							15
16							16
17							17
18							18
19							19
20							20
21							21
22							22
23	PAGE ___ OF ___ CREATION DATE TOTALS ➡						23

50 PAYER NAME	51 HEALTH PLAN ID	52 REL INFO	53 ASG BEN	54 PRIOR PAYMENTS	55 EST. AMOUNT DUE	56 NPI	
A						57 OTHER PRV ID	A
B							B
C							C

58 INSURED'S NAME	59 P.REL	60 INSURED'S UNIQUE ID	61 GROUP NAME	62 INSURANCE GROUP NO.	
A					A
B					B
C					C

63 TREATMENT AUTHORIZATION CODES	64 DOCUMENT CONTROL NUMBER	65 EMPLOYER NAME	
A			A
B			B
C			C

66 DX	67	A	B	C	D	E	F	G	H	68
		I	J	K	L	M	N	O	P	Q

69 ADMIT DX	70 PATIENT REASON DX a b c	71 PPS CODE	72 ECI	73

74 PRINCIPAL PROCEDURE CODE DATE	a. OTHER PROCEDURE CODE DATE	b. OTHER PROCEDURE CODE DATE	75	76 ATTENDING NPI	QUAL
				LAST	FIRST
c. OTHER PROCEDURE CODE DATE	d. OTHER PROCEDURE CODE DATE	e. OTHER PROCEDURE CODE DATE		77 OPERATING NPI	QUAL
				LAST	FIRST
80 REMARKS	81CC a b c d			78 OTHER NPI	QUAL
				LAST	FIRST
				79 OTHER NPI	QUAL
				LAST	FIRST

UB-04 CMS-1450   APPROVED OMB NO. 0938-0997   NUBC National Uniform Billing Committee   THE CERTIFICATIONS ON THE REVERSE APPLY TO THIS BILL AND ARE MADE A PART HEREOF.

Although individual payers have different requirements of when to use the institutional vs. the professional claim forms, institutional claims are intended mostly for facility and supply reimbursement services rather than professional services. That includes room charges, emergency room charges, lab fees, surgery and recovery room charges, diagnostic tests, rehabilitation, supplies, etc. However, charges for specialists, surgeons, radiologists, anesthesiologists, and others involved in the patient's care are not usually included in the hospital claim; instead, they are billed separately using the professional claims form, even though the services were rendered in an institution. Institutional claims are filed by the following types of providers.

- Inpatient Hospitals or Acute Care facilities
- Outpatient Hospital departments/Emergency Rooms
- Skilled Nursing Homes
- Home Health Agencies
- Intermediate Care Facilities
- Clinics
- Hospice Facilities
- Ambulatory Surgery Centers
- Residential Facilities
- Durable Medical Equipment agencies
- Behavioral, Psychiatric and Drug/Alcohol Treatment Centers
- Sub-acute and Long Term Care facilities
- Stand-Alone Ambulatory Surgery Centers

For data analysis purposes, the information elements on the claim form (referred to as Field Locators, or "FL") can be logically grouped into seven categories based on content. Fields of the same category are not necessarily located adjacent to other related fields, but sometimes are scattered almost randomly on the form. Institutional claims follow the general theme that claims involve the patient, provider, physician, payer, medical, visit, and charge information. The following section describes the field locator groups and their data elements.

The purpose of the discussion in this section is not to provide guidance for implementing institutional claims solutions. It is intended to highlight the importance of certain data elements found in institutional claims and their importance to data users with respect to patient data analysis only.

Provider Information - The provider in institutional claims may be any of the previously mentioned facilities. The physician may also be a provider in the same episode of care, but only for their own submitted claims. From the analysis standpoint, the provider is always important to the manufacturer when they can be identified by name and location in the data for targeting purposes. Hospital importance can be measured by the number of specific diagnoses and procedures performed. These diagnoses and procedures must fall in markets of interest to the manufacturer, whether they involve hospital drug therapies, or retail pharmacy drug therapies with potential hospitalization episodes.

NOTE: Targeting applications deal mostly with the entire universe of accounts. Hospital claims databases are based on small samples of hospitals. Targeting applications with hospital claims databases have a limited scope or may not be possible. The provider information may be masked in some databases to protect the patient's confidentiality.

Provider Name
Provider Street Address
Provider City, State, Zip
Provider Telephone, Fax, Country Code
Pay-to Name
Pay-to Address
Pay-to City, State, Zip
Federal Tax Number
NPI
Other Provider ID Primary/ Secondary/Tertiary

The "Provider Name" refers to the institution providing the services while the "Pay-To" entity is the legal entity affiliated with the provider that accepts the payment for the services. The "Federal Tax ID" is unique to the provider, and is sometimes useful in cross-referencing data from different sources. The "Other Provider ID" is the ID assigned to the provider by the payer. There can be up to three "Other Provider IDs," one for each of the payers listed on the claim. With the implementation of the NPI numbers, there is a concerted effort to transition all provider IDs to NPI as the key identifier for any provider in claims processing. The NPI is facility-specific, with each of a provider's multiple facilities assigned their own IDs. All "Other Provider IDs" will eventually diminish in importance.

Physician Information - Similar to pharmacy claims, the physician is also present in the institutional claims. The physician's information is provided for reference purposes only in institutional claims. Physicians are usually reimbursed separately for their hospital services by submitting a claim on the CMS-1500 professional claims form. Because of their importance as key decision makers (when visible in the data) physicians are of interest in data analysis. The physician information on the UB-04 is important to the manufacturer, mostly for targeting purposes and referral pattern analysis. Physician targeting based on partial account universe is subject to the same considerations as the provider targeting above.

The physician section identifies up to four professionals involved in the care of the patient. They include the attending, operating, and two other additional professionals. These physicians may be hospital-salaried staff or independent practitioners.

Attending – NPI/QUAL/ID
Attending – Last/First
Operating – NPI/QUAL/ID
Operating – Last/First
Other ID – QUAL/NPI/QUAL/ID
Other ID – Last/First
Other ID – QUAL/NPI/QUAL/ID
Other ID – Last/First

The "Attending" physician has the overall responsibility for the patient's care, while the "Operating" physician is responsible for performing the main surgical procedures. Other providers listed may include the physician who referred the patient for treatment, an operating physician who performs a secondary surgical procedure, or a rendering physician who performs non-surgical procedures.

Physicians must be identified with their NPI. "Other IDs" include the State License, UPIN, DEA, Provider Commercial Numbers, etc., and are indicated by the "ID Qualifier" field. Data vendors maintain cross-reference tables with many ID types. The "Provider Type Qualifier" identifies the role of any physicians other than the attending and operating. Values of "DN," "ZZ," and "82" indicate the Referring, Other Operating, and Rendering providers, respectively.

Tip: Conventionally, the attending physician is thought to be the diagnosing professional and the operating to be the physician associated with the major procedure. In reality, during a multiple-day stay, it is possible that a patient may have several diagnoses and procedures performed by multiple physicians—not just the attending and operating. With the limitation of four physicians per claim, not all of the physicians may be listed. Nevertheless, if one can accept the first premise, one could then use the data to identify and rank physicians by their number of diagnoses and procedures. Given that the visibility of the physician's influence in the hospital is limited and difficult to gauge, this may be a worthwhile approach.

NOTE: The physician's information may be encrypted in some databases, mainly in payer and employer-sourced databases. An encrypted ID is used to reference the physician longitudinally in data analysis.

Patient & Insured Information - The information in this section is subject to strict HIPAA confidentiality guidelines, and although many fields are encrypted or may not be carried on to the database, the information here is also absolutely ·essential to the longitudinality of the patient history. The patient encryption in institutional claims is consistent with the encryption in professional and pharmacy claims. Any necessary patient attributes like Patient Identifier, and Name must be encrypted with the Patient Birth Year and Month, and Sex unencrypted.

With hospital claims, which are far fewer in number than professional and pharmacy claims, the data may be subject to additional patient privacy considerations. In cases where geographic and age cohorts include too few patients, data may be rolled up to larger patient groups. For example, patients of an age greater than eighty five may be grouped to the same age group, as opposed to ten-year age cohorts. Similarly, patients in a 5-digit zip code may be rolled up to the 3-digit zip code. The Insured's information does not bear any relevance to the longitudinality of the data or importance to the analysis and may be ignored.

Patient Name – Identifier	
Patient Name	
Patient Address - Street	
Patient Address - City	
Patient Address - State	
Patient Address - Zip	
Patient Address – County Code	
Patient Birthdate	
Patient Sex	
Insured's Name - Primary/ Secondary/ Tertiary	Occurs up to 3 times
Patient's Relationship - Primary/ Secondary/ Tertiary	Occurs up to 3 times
Insured's Unique ID - Primary/ Secondary/ Tertiary	Occurs up to 3 times
Insurance Group Name - Primary/ Secondary/ Tertiary	Occurs up to 3 times
Insurance Group Number - Primary/ Secondary/ Tertiary	Occurs up to 3 times
Employer Name - Primary/ Secondary/ Tertiary	Occurs up to 3 times

For payer and employer-sourced databases, the cross-referencing of pharmacy and institutional claims is not necessary. The "Patient Identifier" is the consistent identification of the patient in all claims. Provider and claims switch databases must cross-reference the patient's pharmacy, professional and institutional claims. The "Patient Birthdate" is altered but the month and year are preserved and used to calculate the patient's age. The patient age is in reference to the episode of care, not the present age of the patient. Age and gender are essential elements to patient cohort analysis, because age and gender groups often behave differently in a clinical setting. The patient's 3-digit or 5-digit zip code is usually visible in the data. Geographic disease prevalence, regional treatment patterns, and costs are relevant in data analysis.

The Insured's information on the form is specific to a payer for the as many as three payers listed. The "Insurance Group Name" and "Insurance Group Number" along with the "Payer Name" and "Health Plan ID" fields are useful in identifying the primary medical plan for payer data analysis.

NOTE: Medicare and Medicaid coverage (excluding Managed Medicare, Managed Medicaid, and Part-D) is the same for all patients, and the Insurance Group concept does not apply. It is necessary for all other payers that offer plans with different benefit design options and premiums.

Insurance Payer Information - The payer and plan analysis of pharmacy claims that was of absolute importance to drug manufacturers, as it had a direct impact on product sales, bears less relevance when it comes to hospital reimbursement. From both a clinical and overall burden of illness standpoint, the payer analysis is still relevant to the manufacturer that tries to position drug therapy between other alternatives. With institutional claims, however, because the payer reimburses for drugs indirectly, it is not about formularies, prior authorizations, or co-pays. As a result, data vendors do not usually cross-reference or standardize the payer and plan information in provider and claims switch institutional claims databases the same way they do with pharmacy claims.

Document Control Number	Occurs up to 3 times
Payer Name - Primary/ Secondary/ Tertiary	Occurs up to 3 times
Health Plan ID	Occurs up to 3 times
Treatment Authorization Code - Primary/ Secondary/ Tertiary	Occurs up to 3 times
Release of Information – Primary/ Secondary/ Tertiary	
Assignment of Benefits – Primary/ Secondary/ Tertiary	

The UB-04 allows for up to three payers on the form when the patient is covered by multiple insurance policies in order to coordinate payments between the insurers. For example, a patient over the age of 65 who is covered by Medicare but also covered by the working spouse's employer plan would have two payers listed on the claim form. Payers must be listed in the correct order, with the primary first. This is important because the primary payer carries the main responsibility. Medicare is usually the primary payer, but depending on the employment status of the insured or the spouse, as well as certain conditions met by the employer, Medicare may be a secondary payer.

For each payer, there are a number of associated fields which include the "Payer Name," "Health Plan ID," "Other Provider ID," "Insured's Name" and "Unique ID," "Insurance Group Name" and "Insurance Group Number," "Treatment Authorization Number," "Document Control Number" and "Employer Name." Some of these fields were previously discussed.

The "Document Control Number" is assigned to the claim by the respective payer. It is a kind of case number, and is used to link re-submitted claims to the original submission. When a payer requires pre-authorization for a service, the provider must obtain and report a "Treatment Authorization Code" on the claim. Similar to pharmacy claim, hospital claim prior authorizations are indicative of plan control.

The "Health Plan ID" is a code by which the plan identifies itself to providers. This number will be replaced in the future by the HIPAA National Payer Identifier. This field, together with the "Payer Name" and "Insurance Group Name" and "Group Insurance Group Number," can be used to identify the specific payer and plan.

Tip: Only provider and claims switch-sourced data allow for payer/plan-level analysis. Payer and employer-sourced databases limit the analysis to the plan type level due to payer confidentiality. Payer and employer-sourced data do not reveal the plan identities in the data. Data users should verify the types of charges the database of interest uses in the analysis.

Patient Visit - This section captures various attributes of the patient admission and discharge. These attributes are significant clinically and financially. Clinically, inpatient and outpatient hospitalization and other facility treatments, together with physician visit and drug therapy data, help construct the treatment paths for a disease. Financially, due to managed care pressure to control healthcare costs and payer fixed reimbursement rates regardless of hospitalization days, the length of stay is scrutinized by payers and providers alike and reduced as much as possible.

Patient Control Number
Medical Record Number
Type of Bill
Statement Covers Period – From/Through

Covered Days	
Non-Covered Days	
Coinsurance Days	
Lifetime Reserve Days	
Admission/Start of Care Date	
Admission Hour	
Type of Admission/Visit	
Source of Admission	
Discharge Hour	
Patient Discharge Status	
Condition Codes	Occurs up to 11 times
Accident State	
Occurrence Code/Date	Occurs up to 4 times
Occurrence Span Code/From/Through	Occurs up to 4 times
Responsible Party Name/Address	
Value Code – Code	Occurs up to 12 times
Value Code – Value	Occurs up to 12 times

The "Patient Control Number" is a unique identifier of the specific visit used for billing purposes. The patient is assigned a "Patient Control Number" with every new visit to a hospital. By contrast, the "Medical Record Number" is a permanent number assigned to a patient's medical history that links successive visit records. They are both internal provider identifiers, with no relevance to data analysis.

The "Type of Bill" field indicates the treatment setting and whether the visit was to an inpatient or outpatient department. There are key differences in the way inpatient and outpatient visits are billed by hospitals, and this indicator is important. The 3-digit "Type of Bill" field provides an easy way of determining the treatment setting. The first digit in the code indicates the type of facility. The second digit, for hospitals, implies an inpatient or outpatient setting, but has other interpretations for other facilities. The third digit indicates if the bill is an original claim, a no-charge claim, a supplemental late charge for an already paid claim, a replacement of a prior claim with a revised one, or a void of a submitted claim. A value of "111" indicates a hospital inpatient visit claim and "131" an outpatient visit claim. Other codes are assigned specifically to provider types filling UB-04 forms, such as Skilled Nursing (21X), Home Health (32X), etc. Most commercial databases include inpatient and outpatient hospital claims with Type of Bill "111" and "131."

The "Statement Covers Period – From/Through" marks the start and end dates of services covered on the bill. For inpatient visits, these dates usually coincide with the admission and discharge dates, and are used to calculate the length of stay. Outpatient visits usually have the same "From" and "Through" dates, but there are exceptions where the patient enters the facility on one date and leaves on another. In other cases, certain payers require a single outpatient bill for an entire period of time that covers a patient's multiple visits to an outpatient department. For example, a physical therapy patient who makes several outpatient visits to a hospital would require a single claim for the entire month. The type and date of charges are listed on the bill. These claims are referred to as "series" accounts.

TIP: From the data standpoint, to properly and longitudinally reflect the patient episodes of care, claims for series accounts should be broken down to each visit.

The "Admission/Start of Care Date" is the actual admission date for inpatient visits or the start date of the episode of care for Home Health services. The "Type of Admission/Visit" indicates the level of severity and urgency of the patient's condition. There are codes for emergency, urgent, elective, trauma, etc.

The "Source of Admission" indicates how the patient was referred to the institution for treatment. For example, a physician's referral, transfer from another facility, emergency room referral, etc. It is also used to indicate if a newborn was delivered normally or with any adverse conditions, such as being premature or sick. The "Patient Discharge Status" indicates whether the patient was discharged home, transferred to a short-term care facility, transferred to a skilled nursing facility, if the patient expired, etc. The "Source of Admission" and "Patient Discharge Status" can be used to analyze admission, discharge, and hospital referral patterns for certain conditions.

The "Condition Codes" are used to indicate special circumstances and events that could potentially affect the processing of the claim. There are dozens of condition codes that vary widely to be easily grouped in predefined categories. However, if a specific code of interest is identified, it could potentially be used as a condition in the patient cohort selection. For example, by using the code "B3," one could limit the cohort to patients with a pregnancy indicator, or use the code "02" for employment-related medical conditions.

The "Occurrence Codes" with their associated "Occurrence Dates" are used to identify chronologically significant events that are relevant to the processing of the billing. Although "Occurrence Codes" cover a great variety of events, use of these codes in data analysis is sparse at best. The codes could potentially be useful in sequencing an event in relation to another milestone date. For example, using code "11" to determine the lapsed time between the "Onset of Symptoms/Illness" and the time of hospitalization.

The "Value Code–Code" and "Value Code–Value" fields are used to quantify certain metrics related to the claim. They provide rates, amounts, quantities, service units, length of time, weights, etc., as they relate to the appropriate variable being measured; this information includes the number of units of an administered drug, the daily room rate for a private room bed, the number of visits to a rehab center, and the amount of co-insurance.

The "Value Code," "Condition Code," and "Occurrence Code" fields are very rich in terms of content, but difficult to use in data analysis. Unlike variables representing a single dimension with multiple possible values, these variables represent multiple dimensions with multiple values. The many-to-many relationship between dimensions and values further complicates the analysis. One must first determine the desired dimension and then query the data for the specific values. These variables are underutilized in data analysis, and in fact, may not be present in certain patient databases.

Charge Information - This is a key section of the UB-04 form that outlines the charges for a specific episode of care. Like pharmacy claims, however, the claim represents the economics only from the provider side. The more accurate cost figures are the ones that are stated in the remittance advice sent back from the payer. The remittance outlines the payer-allowed and paid amounts. The Allowed amount is usually the amount a payer pays the provider for a service, plus the patient's share of the cost, which may include deductibles, co-pay and co-insurance. The paid amount is the payer's portion of the cost.

Revenue Code
Revenue Code Description
HCPCS/Rates/HIPPS Rate Codes
Service Date
Units of Service
Total Charges
Non-Covered Charges
Prior Payments - Primary/ Secondary/ Tertiary
Estimated Amount Due - Primary/ Secondary/ Tertiary

Hospital charges are based on "Revenue Codes." Revenue codes describe the category of the product or services rendered and are used for both inpatient and outpatient claims. However, inpatient and outpatient claims use revenue codes differently. Inpatient charges are summarized and rolled up under the applicable revenue codes. Outpatient charges, on the other hand, are itemized and detailed to include all of the services, drugs, and supplies. For example, in the inpatient setting, there would be a single laboratory revenue code listed for any number of lab tests performed during the stay summarizing the charges for all tests. For outpatient claims, each laboratory charge would be listed separately, along with the revenue code and the applicable HCPCS code and date of service. Revenue codes are four digit codes with the first three digits describing the charge category and the fourth digit qualifying a more specific case. For example, code "0360" refers to the general classification of operating room charges. Code "0361" refers to operating room charges for a minor surgery.

Even though providers use revenue codes to report the charges, Medicare and other payers use diagnosis-related groups (DRGs) to calculate the reimbursement amount. These payers reimburse a fixed amount for the entire hospitalization based on the most appropriate DRG, regardless of the resources consumed by the patient's care. A DRG is based on the average resources to treat patients of certain diagnoses, ages, genders, co-morbid conditions, and complications. Medicare calculates the DRG amounts by comparing the cost of care for similar claims with the same length of stay. Cost data is collected annually by Medicare from health care institutions and takes into consideration geographic labor cost and cost of living indexes. A hospital may receive an add-on payment for a DRG if it treats a high-percentage of low-income patients. This add-on is known as the disproportionate share hospital (DSH) adjustment. Additionally, approved teaching hospitals receive a percentage add-on payment for each case. This amount varies depending on the ratio of residents to beds. Exceptions are made and additional payments are provided for outlier cases with unusually large length of stays and charges. DRGS were developed as part of Medicare's inpatient prospective payment system (IPPS) and were intended to encourage providers to become more efficient and cost effective with their services in order to reduce the length of stay and turnaround time for certain services. Currently, there are over five hundred defined DRG codes. Certain services and institutions are exempt from this reimbursement method. The hospital's coding staff apply the most applicable DRG code and report it on the claim in the "PPS" field.

The "HCPCS/Rates" is a key field, and provides either the HCPCS code for outpatient claims or a charge rate for inpatient claims. Inpatient claims do not use HCPCS codes, but instead use the "Procedure Codes" discussed in the Diagnosis/Procedures section. In the case of an administered drug with a specific Level II HCPCS code in an outpatient department, a Q or J code will describe the drug used.

NOTE: This is another key difference between inpatient and outpatient claims that highlights a major limitation with inpatient claims data: inpatient claims do not allow visibility to drug utilization, which is of great importance to drug manufacturers. Even though outpatient claims itemize the HCPCS Level II drug code, many codes are used to describe therapeutic equivalent drugs, and, even though one can identify the class, the specific brand may not be identifiable.

The "Service Date" is used in outpatient claims only. It was intended to record the date of service in "series" accounts for repeat visits to an outpatient department, but it is used even in non-series claims as well.

The "Units of Service" provide a quantifiable measure of the services or products. The type of units measured varies by product or service. It may represent a rate expressed in dollars, the quantity of drug administered, number of room days, number of treatments, etc.

The "Total Charges" are specific to a "Revenue Code" and include both covered and non-covered amounts. The "Non-Covered Charges" are also specific to "Revenue Codes." The claim grand totals for "Total Charges" and "Non-Covered Charges" are provided on line 23 of the last page of the UB-04, with a "Revenue Code" of "0001."

The total amount is the provider's reimbursable cost estimate of the claim. The payer may adjust that amount and will advise the provider of the reimbursed amount based on contracted rates and the patient's responsibility. If there is supplemental insurance, the institution will bill any other payers for non-reimbursed and non-covered amounts before it attributes the balance to the patient's responsibility amount.

The "Prior Payments" field is used for coordination of benefits. It lists the amount previously paid by the patient or by another payer. The "Estimated Amount Due" reflects the expected reimbursement amount net of any "Prior Payments". It can be either the same as the "Total Charges" or the balance of any unpaid charges from the primary payer to the secondary.

Diagnosis/Procedure Information - This section captures some of the most important aspects of institutional care. It provides the basis for epidemiological and treatment data in the institutional setting. Institutional diagnosis and procedure data, together with the physician's office diagnoses and procedures, and pharmacy drug utilization data, is the basis for disease treatment pattern analysis.

Principal Diagnosis Code & Present on Admission Indicator	
Admitting Diagnosis Code & Present on Admission Indicator	
Other Diagnosis & Present on Admission Indicator	Occurs up to 17 times
Present on Admission Indicator	
Patient's Reason for Visit Code	Occurs up to 3 times

PPS Code	
External Cause of Injury Code	Occurs up to 3 times
HCPCS Codes	
Principal Procedure Code/Date	
Other Procedure Code/Date	Occurs up to 5 times

The UB-04 provides space for one "Principal Diagnosis," one "Admitting," and seventeen "Other Diagnosis Codes." The "Principal Diagnosis Code" describes the primary cause of the treatment and is determined subsequently to admission. The principal diagnosis might be different from the admitting diagnosis. This is because the "Admitting Diagnosis Code" is based on initial judgment from early findings and symptoms at the time of admission, and as such, has the potential for an initial misdiagnosis. All "Other Diagnosis Codes" for comorbid conditions that affect the treatment, either present at the time of the admission or acquired thereafter, are also listed. The "Present on Admission Indicator" is the eighth digit of principal, admitting, and other diagnosis codes that indicates the existence of the condition at the time of the patient's admission to an inpatient facility, or if the condition was acquired as a result of the hospital stay. The indicator is used for national statistics purposes in the realm of public health reporting.

When external causes such as injuries, poisoning, etc. are the reason for the visit, or when they occur during treatment, the "External Cause of Injury" (ECI) diagnosis codes are used to describe them.

The "Patient's Reason for Visit" diagnosis codes are determined and reported based on the patient's stated reason at the time of an outpatient visit for seeking treatment. This information may bear relevance to the adjudication of a claim. Both the admitting and patient's reason for visit diagnoses are not considered in a cohort selection based on diagnosis codes.

The "Prospective Payment System (PPS) Code" is used to identify the applicable DRG code for reimbursement purposes when Medicare is the payer, or for when the payer is contracted to reimburse a provider based on DRGs.

TIP: Providers sometimes list as a primary diagnosis the one that will result in the highest reimbursement. The principal diagnosis is likely to be the reason for the principal or other procedures, but not necessarily so. For analytical purposes and for selecting patient cohorts, the selection criteria may not be limited to the principal diagnosis. For that matter, the same is true for procedures.

The "Principal," "Other Procedure Codes," and their corresponding "Dates" are designated to describe up to six of the most important medical procedures performed on a patient during an inpatient stay for an episode of care. There are two types of procedure codes: the HCPCS and the ICD-9 Volume III codes. The HCPCS Level I and II codes are used to identify procedures performed in outpatient settings. The ICD-9 codes are used by inpatient facilities. The UB-04 form has designated separate fields for inpatient and outpatient codes. The HCPCS codes are populated in the "HCPCS/RATE/HIPPS/CODE" field while the ICD-9 codes are populated in the "Principal Procedure" and "Other Procedure" fields.

Advantages of Claims Data

Claims data is the most prolific, abundant, and easily collectible type of patient data that can be accessed through multiple sources: namely, providers, claims switches, payers, and employers. The claims process is such that a high concentration of data passing through only a few traffic points will create an efficient way to collect the data.

The underlying reason for this inherent efficiency is the technology used and the level of automation implemented across the parties involved in the claims process. This includes software implemented at the provider sites for coding and electronic claim submission, the routing process and switching technology to get the claim from the provider to the payer (which is handled by the claims clearinghouses), the conversion from paper to electronic claims, and the claims adjudication software on the payer end.

A major advantage with claims data is the existence of standards for processing paper form or electronic claims. Standards keep data disparity from different collection points to a minimum and allow for the aggregation and standardization of large amounts of data with relatively little effort. That holds true for data both across collection points of the same source type, and across the source types themselves. It is relatively easy to integrate data from providers, claims switches, employers, and payers in order to form a claims database. In the best-case scenario, the least common denominator of data elements will be the standard itself.

The standards also assure the existence of a finite number of data elements. That in itself is important because it provides a range of what is possible with the data and defines the scope of solutions. As we will see with EMR data, another important type of patient database, that range and scope is difficult to define; consequently, it limits the data's predictability.

While other patient data types capture solely the medical perspectives of care, claims data is unique in capturing both the medical and financial perspectives.

Claims data is the only data type to capture the cost of care across the spectrum of healthcare settings: pharmacy, physician practice and institution.

Limitations of Claims Data

Healthcare claims serve financial purposes, and therefore, the strengths of the data in that area are easily understood. Claims need to include just enough of the relevant medical information about the products and services rendered in order to be adjudicated. As a result, the amount of clinical data they contain is limited. Consequently, while claims data sufficiently address financial applications, they lack some important aspects necessary in clinical data analysis.

In some cases, the most essential clinical information (namely, the diagnosis) is not present. By design, pharmacy data lacks the diagnosis indication for the dispensed scripts. Although the diagnosis for pharmacy claims can be retrieved from the corresponding professional claims, it is subject to limitations in the cross-referencing between the two.

It was mentioned above that the existence of standards minimizes the disparity of data from different sources. However, data elements are usually subject to restricted use by the data sources, thereby causing an induced type of disparity. In addition, the varying requirements of payers with respect to submitted information for claims adjudication often results in data fields being populated inconsistently. The purpose of standards, in the case of claims, is to define the maximum scope of the data, rather than the minimum requirements.

Claims data does not lend itself well to measuring medical outcomes, either. Even though the claim documents the utilization of care over time, it does not capture directly its effects. Thus, the cause and effect relationships are not evident in the data. Here again, the analyst must look for subsequent evidence in the patient's history to identify possible outcomes. For example, one may determine if a therapy associated with a disease stage had an effect by looking for evidence of a different therapy associated with a later stage of the disease.

Another limitation with claims data is the lack of staging information that would clearly identify the patient's disease progression. The data does generally capture the patient's diagnosis. However, from the therapy standpoint, the diagnosis is not sufficient—treatments are often tied to specific stages of the disease. To address this limitation of claims data, analysts have to indirectly determine the disease stage through the association of current treatments to a disease stage based on empirical knowledge.

In cases where the diagnosis was absent from the pharmacy claims but the drug utilization was captured in great detail, the opposite almost holds true with respect to institutional claims, and to some extent with professional claims. There, the

101

diagnosis is available, but not necessarily will the drug therapy be, too. Because institutional inpatient claims are collections of bundled services rather than itemized lists of units of products and services, the drug is usually disguised under the procedure. With all outpatient claims, drugs with a J-Code are visible in the data. However, the description may lack clarity, in which case it may imply one of many drugs.

Despite the fact that the claims process is automated to a great degree, and that software is widely adopted, the process itself is such that it causes certain incompatibilities between the different claim types. One obvious difference is the timing of claim submission and adjudication. We saw how pharmacy claims are adjudicated instantly as they are submitted; therefore, both the claim and the remittance advice transactions are immediately available for reporting. Professional claims, on the other hand, have both a longer submission and adjudication timetable, depending on both how promptly the office is submitting claims and the how long the payer's claim backlog is. Hospital claims are subject to similar limitations. As a result, a patient's recent episodes of care are partially documented in the claims data at the end of a reporting period. To close the timing gap, some sources will report submitted rather than reimbursed claims, or they may lag the data by several months.

Lastly, while the data structures of claims data are rather simple, working with claims data is not. Claims data requires the implementation of complex business rules to mine it adequately. That is partly due to some of the limitations discussed here and partly due to the extensive coding used. The lack of enrollment and staging data, for example, would require algorithms to extract it from other relevant pieces of information. The complexity of the data and the lack of end-user experience contribute to high costs and client dependence on the vendor's trained professional staff.

Prescription Data

Perhaps the oldest and closest type of syndicated product to patient data still in the market today is pharmacy prescription data. Prescription data comes from the same source of data as one of the most prominent patient data types: pharmacy claims data. In fact, in some instances, the vendors may use the same collected data for both claims and prescription databases, but with the prescription data aggregated and presented differently.

Prescription data comes from patient level pharmacy transactions. In early versions, the patient attributes were stripped and the data was aggregated at the prescribing physician; these records were counting the number of times a practitioner prescribed a product during a time period and the prescribed quantity.

In an attempt to find a tool that would identify prescribing physicians for targeting purposes, the data was presented in a way that took the focus away from the patient and made the physician the central figure. Traditionally, the legacy prescription data products lacked the longitudinal aspect of the patient. The data was a snapshot in time, rather than a time-sequenced set of events that revolved around the patient.

Recent versions of the prescription data products, even though they are still aggregations at the physician level, include some patient dimension breakdowns such as age and gender. In addition, they offer a longitudinal perspective, breaking down the prescription activity to new, continuing, and switched, relative to the patient's treatment status from the previous reporting period.

Medicare Standard Analytical File

The Medicare patient population is often of interest in research projects because of the high prevalence of chronic diseases in that age group. Medicare publishes its claims data in the Standard Analytical Files (SAF). The files are produced out of Medicare's repository of claims, the National Claims History (NCH) file. The NCH file captures all inpatient and outpatient claims. The SAF files include final action claims. These are non-rejected claims for which a payment has been made, all disputes have been resolved, and final adjustments to original claims have been made. The files list multiple claims for the same episode separately. The files are produced annually with quarterly updates.

The institutional SAF files include claims for inpatient, outpatient, SNF, hospice, and HHA from 1989. The non-institutional file includes Part-B claims from physicians, suppliers and laboratory services. Because Medicare did not offer a pharmacy benefit until 2006, currently there are no Medicare Part-D files. Any future Part-D files would start with the year 2006. The 100% SAF files include all of the claims, while the 5% SAF beneficiary samples are subsets of the claims based on a selection method that takes records with 05, 20, 45, 70, or 95 in position 8 and 9 of the patient's Health Insurance Claim (HIC) number. The HIC is the beneficiary's unique identification number: usually, their a nine-digit social security number (SSN) and a two-character code signifying the beneficiary's relationship to the primary holder of the associated SSN, though there are some exceptions.

The 5% beneficiary sample data came about by necessity due to the enormously large Part-B claims data file. Medicare dealt with that by selecting a 5% beneficiary sample from the Part-B claims file and matching them with the institutional claims of the same beneficiaries. Medicare allows researchers to match their own patient cohorts to claims data from the SAF files by submitting a custom list of patients.

That is called the "finder file," and it includes patient identifying information like name, date of birth, gender, SSNs, and HICs, if available.

The Medicare SAF files are compatible with other claims databases because they are based on the same UB-92, CMS-1500 and ASCI X12N electronic standards for submitted claims. Samples of Medicare claims are captured in provider and claims switch-sourced patient databases, and are representative of the Medicare population. Some Medicare claims are captured even in payer and employer-sourced databases when the claim involves coordination of benefits with Medicare as the primary payer. The Medicare sample in these databases is not significant or representative, however.

Medicare offers different versions of its claims data. The Denominator file is a type of enrollment file that contains basic demographic data on each beneficiary enrolled during the particular coverage year. The Research Identifiable Files (RIFs) are un-encrypted claims files requiring a rigorous application and review process to obtain. The Beneficiary Encrypted Files (BEFs), are similar to RIFs in content, but some patient identifying fields are encrypted. These files are easier to obtain that RIFs. One limitation of the BEFs is that patients whose HIC changed during the data extraction period are not cross-referenced, and their claims in the BEF file will appear as claims of different patients. Medicare also produces high-level, aggregated Public Use Files (PUFs), downloadable for free or a small fee. Medicare also publishes the MedPAR file, which is discussed in the next chapter.

The SAF files are useful by themselves for analysis of the Medicare population. There are certain restrictions, however, related to the use of the files. CMS requires that the data must be used only in health-related research, evaluation, or epidemiology projects. CMS does not allow use of the data in commercial applications such as a manufacturer's sales and marketing activities. Manufacturers may still qualify for access to the files for science-based applications, however.

CMS requires a written request outlining the purpose of the data need, description and methodology of data use, and a list of specific data requirements and selection criteria. In addition, it requires a study protocol and an outline of the scientific methodology to be used in the data analysis. The person submitting the request must also provide evidence of funding and sign a data use agreement. From the submitted information, CMS will determine if the RIF file is required or if an alternative encrypted file might meet the requirements instead. In addition, it determines if the privacy of the patients is adequately protected and if the study can be reasonably performed with the data before it approves the request.

Chapter 3
Hospital Databases

Charge Master-Level Data

The charge description master (CDM) or charge master system is a very vital component of a hospital's billing software. It catalogs all billable products and services provided by the hospital, along with their associated pricing. The painstaking cataloging includes everything from gauze to medical procedures, and is essential in order to attribute costs to a specific patient visit. Typically, a charge master system numbers from a few thousand to tens of thousands of entries.

Charge master entries, where applicable, include information beyond the typical item number, description, unit of measure, and price, such as a department code to charge the item to the appropriate revenue center within the hospital. Listed procedures are mapped to the appropriate CPT and revenue codes that appear on the UB-04 bill.

The pricing of the items in the charge master is set using various methods. For purchased items, the pricing method is usually the application of a markup. Services are more difficult to price because they involve both supplies and labor. In the case of a procedure, supplies and the hospital's labor rates are used to calculate an average cost.

Alternatively, a hospital may use benchmark data from a group of hospitals to set such pricing. It may choose, for example, to set the price of a procedure to the average price of a given percentile from a group of hospitals, thus avoiding the complex process of determining costs. The problem with this method is that the procedure may not be profitable at the averaged price if the hospital's cost structure is significantly different than that of the hospitals used in the benchmark data.

To keep the charge master current with price updates, the hospital typically assigns a "charge master team" to the task. The periodic update of the pricing is vital to the hospital to stay current with the cost increases of supplies and services in order to remain profitable. However, with the thousands of products in the table, the task of updating such a database is not easy. Updates to the product master are made either by applying the same price increase uniformly across the board, or by using cost accounting and adjusting the cost of components within the service.

A hospital records the charges for inpatient and outpatient visits at the lowest level, accounting for every item used in the patient's care. However, as mentioned in an earlier section, the actual hospital billing is summarized on the UB-04 form. Given the limited use of the itemization of the products and services in billing and reimbursement, the charge master's utility is generally relegated to dictating cost only. The hospital not only uses the data to analyze its own cost structure, but also for required reporting to Medicare or other state and federal reporting.

NOTE: The industry refers frequently to charge master data to denote patient-level charges itemized at the charge master entry level. That data is not stored in the charge master, as the term might imply, but instead is stored in a separate data table of the billing system. The charge master is simply a pricing table.

For patient data analysis, the itemized listing of products and services holds special importance, particularly for the manufacturer, given the lack of drug utilization data in inpatient hospital claims. The lack of that data prevents analysts from completing the patient's treatment profile across therapy modes. While the surgical and radiological therapies are visible in the data, the inpatient hospital drug therapy is not. Similarly, the analyst has visibility to drug therapy from pre and post-hospitalization treatment, but not to the drug therapy used during the stay.

The charge master-level patient data comes to complete that picture by providing the missing hospital drug utilization. When linked to claims data for the same hospitals, it forms an expanded claims database that includes drug utilization. Ultimately, the linking of the data to professional and pharmacy claims creates a very powerful database.

NOTE: Outpatient hospital drug utilization is available through both the hospital outpatient claims and the charge master-level data. Current charge master-level databases are made up of smaller hospital panels as opposed to hospital claims databases, and therefore a claims database is not fully expanded with charge master-level detail. The addition is, however, significant enough for data applications.

There is a key limitation with charge master-level detail data: in most cases, the references to drugs in the data are such that a clear distinction between brands and manufacturers cannot be made for drugs of the same molecule. Manufacturers are interested in quantifying the usage of their own drugs and comparing that amount to the competition; this lack of specificity impedes such analyses.

The reasons for the lack of specificity are rather easily understood. On one end, the physician making treatment decisions determines the appropriate drug for the therapy, while at the other end, the pharmacist tries to acquire the drug at a favorable price. It is usually in the best interests of the hospital that these decisions are made independently; when the physician issues an order for the administration of a drug, the pharmacist will match that request with the drug ordered by the physician or an equivalent based on inventory. The lack of clarifying information, such as the NDC code of the drug, results in the ambiguous reference of the product in the data.

This process exposes the different dynamics in the physician's influence in the retail versus the hospital setting. In the retail setting, barring any formulary limitations, the physician may unequivocally make use of the no-substitution flag on the script and assure the dispensing of a specific brand. The physician's choice or preference is limited in the hospital setting. While targeting office-based physicians has a direct impact on product sales on the retail side, on the hospital side, the action is more about pharmacy contracting than it is about physician targeting.

In terms of managed care, the outpatient side is tremendously important. However, on the hospital side, payers are not billed directly for drugs. In fact, they do not have any visibility to drug utilization. There, payers have more control over the type of therapy used and may choose to reimburse for one but not another, or even choose the order of therapies given. However, for a reimbursable procedure, payers are rather indifferent about the pharmacist's drug choices—the reimbursement is usually the same, regardless of the drug used.

When the charge master-level patient data is linked to outpatient and professional claims, the data shows the drug therapy the patient was on before, during and after hospitalization, and in the process, exposes any drug switching. Another key demonstration lies in the variances in hospital drug treatment between inpatient and outpatient. Often, because inpatient and outpatient reimbursement rates vary, they affect drug utilization. This holds especially true for inpatient visits, given that the hospital is often reimbursed at a fixed rate by DRG. The hospital often manages its costs by controlling drug dosing. Outpatient drug use is usually not as restrictive, due to a more relaxed reimbursement scheme. The data can also be used to demonstrate the effect of appropriate drug dosing on the hospital length of stay.

The recording of charges by department is a key feature of the charge master. It allows analysts to trace the source of services, the progression of care, and the key departments of the hospital to a particular therapy. For example, the data shows the role of the ER prior to hospitalization for a disease, how often ICU services are involved, the extent of the pharmacy and lab use, etc.

Charge master detail is even more valuable when it is time stamped or sequenced. Internally, the hospital systems that track the patient's care usually record the date and time of events. However, that information may not be provided to data vendors. The sequencing allows analysts to better understand how care is given and the role that a hospital's treatment protocols affect that care. Charge master databases vary in this respect. Ideally, time stamping is most desirable, with simple sequencing serving as a good compromise.

Medicare Provider Analysis and Review File

The Medicare Provider Analysis and Review (MedPAR) is a patient discharge data file produced from Medicare's National Claims History file. Unlike the SAF files, the MedPAR file is not a claim-level file but a stay-level file. That is, multiple claims for the same patient admission are consolidated into a single record. Each patient stay or discharge may have more than one final action claim associated with it. This occurs for approximately 5-20% of the inpatient stays depending on the type of inpatient facility: short or long term.

The MedPAR files contain information for 100% of the Medicare inpatient beneficiaries. There is a MedPAR file for each of long-stay hospitals, short-stay hospitals, and skilled nursing facilities (SNFs). There are no MedPAR files for outpatient beneficiaries. Below is a list of some key data elements listed in the MedPAR files.

Claim Account Number
Patient Demographics
Admission Date
Admission Type Code
Discharge Date
Length of State
Discharge Status
Discharge Destination Code

Provider Number	
Beneficiary Deductibles and Coinsurance	
Total Charge Amount	
Total Covered Charge Amount	
Primary Payer Amount	
Medicare Payment Amount	
DRG Outlier Payment Amount	
Inpatient Disproportionate Amount	
Revenue Center Charges	One per revenue center
Use of Services Indicators	
Primary and Secondary Diagnoses	Occurs up to 10 times
Primary and Secondary Procedures	Occurs up to 6 times
Procedure Dates	Occurs up to 6 times
DGR Code	
:	

A "Claim Account Number" is a unique number assigned to the Medicare beneficiary. Patient demographics are provided for patient cohort analysis by age, sex and geographic location. The "Admission Type," "Length of Stay," and "Discharge Status" are characteristically important data elements of discharge databases, along with the procedures, diagnoses, and DRG codes. The provider, a facility in this case, can be identified only with an encoded facility identifier. The type of facility distinction, such as teaching hospitals, disproportionate share hospitals, etc., is essential to the analysis. The MedPAR file does not include any physician information.

Since the MedPAR files are sourced from the claims files, they summarize data for all services rendered during the stay. Charges in the MedPAR files are summarized from the revenue code level in the UB-04 form to the revenue center. Revenue centers are much fewer in number and are more general categories, with each represented as a field in the file layout.

There are no outpatient or Part-B MedPAR files available, and as such, MedPAR is inadequate for tracking patients across the care continuum. The MedPAR files are best suited for Medicare inpatient discharge analysis and statistics. They have an advantage over the SAF files when the intent of the analysis is the stay, rather than the specific claim, due to the fact that the files have consolidated multiple claims for the same stay into a single record.

Discharge data is important to the manufacturer. However, the manufacturer's objective in analyzing the data is usually to examine the broader market, which is hardly Medicare alone. The MedPAR file is very important, albeit indirectly. Its data is incorporated in larger commercial discharge databases in order to provide a more comprehensive view of the market.

Hospital Discharge Data

Hospital discharge data is a data category that focuses on summarizing hospital stays. MedPAR data is a good example of a discharge dataset that is limited to Medicare patients only, yet representative of all Medicare patients. More comprehensive databases incorporate Medicare, Medicaid, third party, and cash patients from the broadest set of hospitals, and although national statistics are often the desired level of detail, these databases focus on hospital-level detail.

Discharge data originates in hospital medical claims. This is because claims data includes all the right elements for a discharge, not to mention that it is easily available and is sometimes already in use for other purposes. In that respect, discharge data is a byproduct of claims data. As such, and similar to claims data, discharge data is concerned with admission and discharge status and length of stay, diagnoses and procedures, charge data, and payment types.

Discharge data is useful to various user types. Manufacturers use the data to size their inpatient market opportunity for an indication by using the overall number of relevant diagnoses and procedures performed at each hospital as a proxy. Discharge data is also useful in targeting applications, as it identifies high-ranking hospitals based on diagnosis and procedure volume. This technique is useful when other metrics like drug sales to hospitals do not adequately reflect the hospital's importance. For providers, it serves as benchmark data for their own performance. It allows them to compare their own metrics (such as length of stay and charge data for specific diagnoses) to industry averages. Case load analysis allows providers to compare their Medicare and private insurance share of patients to other providers. Payers, too, can measure their performance against the competition and contrast private and government payers. National statistics are important to a number of government and private entities.

Commercial discharge databases are compiled mainly through four sources: state hospital associations, non-federal hospitals, Medicare, and VA/DOD hospitals. These databases offer census or projected data for almost all hospitals in the US. The bulk of the data comes from the state hospital associations. A large number of states collect discharge data from all the non-federal hospitals in the state for statistical purposes, which they subsequently make available to data vendors. Vendors partially fill in for the remaining states using claims data collected from hospitals and hospital chains. For all other hospitals in these states, vendors use the Medicare SAF or MedPAR files from CMS to establish a data sample, at the very least. From this partial data, vendors use projections to estimate the totals based on hospital profiles, such as number of beds, admissions, Medicare-to-commercial claims ratios, etc. Finally, the federal hospital data for all states made available through the Veterans Administration (VA) may be used by some vendors to complete the data set. The slide below shows a typical discharge report with aggregate information.

Even though discharge data maintains the granularity at the patient and visit level, the longitudinal dimension is compromised. Discharge data does not meet all the qualifying dimensions to be considered true patient data. Discharge data is also limited to institutions only, and therefore, it is not suitable for studies across all aspects of care. Discharge data does not include all of the data elements found in hospital claims, either. Also, because it is compiled from numerous sources, it is significantly less timely than claims data. However, it is a less cumbersome dataset; it is easier and faster to work with. That, together with the summary nature of the data, makes discharge data a quicker and less expensive alternative to claims data for certain applications.

Chapter 4
Electronic Medical Records

What are Electronic Medical Records?

Electronic Medical Records (EMR), also known as Electronic Health Records (EHR), are patient-level medical information, and the equivalent of the patient's complete medical chart. Electronic medical records are the result of the systematic electronic recording of patient episodic, longitudinal information in physician's offices, outpatient clinics, and hospitals. The information goes beyond what is captured through claims data. EMR data is the result of the intentional capture of essential details about a patient's care; it does not come into existence in the same inadvertent way as one observes in claims data.

When it comes to a patient's care, every minute detail counts. If it is worth putting on the medical chart, it is valuable information. That detail becomes important "circumstantial evidence" for a professional reviewing the patient's records, or a researcher looking for clues and answers. The reality is that it also represents a lot of information, and much of it will be important only in limited circumstances.

In the physician's practice, where the vast majority of the patient encounters take place, EMR data is still in the early stages of evolution. Driven mostly by economics, the adoption of EMR systems in solo and small group practices has a lot of ground to cover. In terms of the acquisition and maintenance costs of the software, as well as the required effort to input the information, there are numerous

113

drawbacks for the professional. Additionally, even though EMR systems are an elegant solution considering the technological state of the industry, the reality is that the task of managing a disease varies by the diseases themselves. Certain specialties of professionals are more likely to adopt the technology than others based on need. Oncologists, for example, given the complexity of cancer treatments, are good candidates for adopting EMR technology.

Given the unique nature of diseases, EMR systems typically consist of a core applicable to all diseases, with custom functionality for specific specialties built-in in order to capture data elements that are unique to a disease. Similarly, the reporting system is customized to output the unique features. There are EMR systems customized for a number of specialties, including allergy, cardiology, general medicine, pain management, otolaryngology, gastroenterology, internal medicine, OB-GYN, pediatrics, pulmonary, sleep medicine, etc.

One initiative that is aiding the proliferation of EMR software is CMS' Doctor's Office Quality – Information Technology (DOQ-IT) initiative. This initiative was designed to capture observational data from the physician's practice with respect to coronary artery disease, heart failure, diabetes, hypertension, and preventive care. The project requires the electronic transmission of data from EMR systems into the DOQ-IT data warehouse. To accelerate the transition to electronic health systems, CMS offered free assistance to primary care physician practices treating Medicare patients for the assessment, planning, selection, implementation and optimization of EMR, eRx and patient registry systems. Although these initiatives are mainly intended for the benefit of Medicare patients, they benefit the larger patient population and the industry as a whole.

EMR System Functionality

EMR systems are usually not standalone systems, but rather a component of a larger suite of applications that include practice and revenue cycle management systems. The true value of these systems lies in the integration of these components and the complete management of the patient care, which includes setting appointments, recording the visit, billing insurance, and receiving of payments. The functionality of these systems includes electronic charts, radiology and lab ordering services, electronic prescribing directly to the pharmacy, and personal health record communication. Systems may include a patient access module for communication with the professional, as well as a review of their medical and prescription history. Below are some of the standard EMR system components.

- **Patient Record** - EMR systems establish and maintain patient records that are complete with the patient demographic information, such as name, address, sex, age, etc. The patient is identified by system-assigned identifiers in addition to external identifiers such as a third party payer or Medicare-assigned IDs.

- **Patient History** - EMRs capture and manage the patient's history. That includes diagnoses, procedures, medical or surgical problems, and family and social histories. Medical history usually looks for both the presence and absence of certain conditions. Information is captured either directly from the patient by using an input form, or indirectly by using the patient's personal health record, electronic input from another provider, etc. With the proliferation of EMR systems, a patient's history will be soon be transferable electronically across providers.

- **Problem List** - EMRs maintain lists of any current and historical problems or diagnoses by date. Problems are usually identified as chronic or acute and have medication, lab orders, and clinical notes associated with them. Systems can identify specific visits for specific diagnoses. The information is coded with the appropriate clinical code sets.

- **Medication List** - EMR systems maintain the patient's current and historical lists of prescribed and dispensed medications. Lists are coded with standard abbreviations and are complete with product names, dates, doses, administration routes, signas, dispense amounts, refills and the associated diagnoses. Medication lists include both prescription and over-the-counter products. The history may include therapy start and renewal dates. Communication with the pharmacy allows the capture of fill notifications.

- **Allergy and Adverse Affects List** - These systems allow users to maintain lists of medications, immunizations, and other agents the patient is allergic to. The information is used for cross-checking prescribed drugs to prevent adverse reactions. They also capture non-drug allergic agents, such as environmental and food allergens.

- **Clinical Encounters** - EMRs may be used to document provider-patient encounters. The systems associate each encounter with diagnoses and record the healthcare delivered during the encounter. This includes the administration or supply of medications and immunizations, with complete documentation of dosage, time, route of administration, site, product, manufacturer, etc. Current or prior reactions to immunization are noted. The systems provide a flexible means of capturing the data, both in structured form (by using templates and surveys) and free-text form. The users can choose elements manually, select from pick lists, or dictate for a later transcription by using voice recognition.

- **Electronic Charting** - EMR systems provide the functionality to create and manage documents and notes and associate them with the patient diagnoses, problems and encounters. These may include vital signs like blood pressure, heart rate, respiratory rate, physiological data like height and weight, and other clinical data elements, such as peak expiratory flow rate, lesion size, severity of pain, etc. Notes are created both in free-text form and as structured, codified input that can be searched, indexed and filtered. Structured input uses industry standard coding sets such as MEDCIN, SNOMED CT, ICD-9, CPT, NDC, etc. The systems also provide the ability to capture external clinical documents, including scanned documents, faxes, consultant reports, referral authorizations, provider-to-provider communication, patient communication of clinical nature, electronic lab results from an external source or lab equipment interface, radiology images, image documents, etc. Systems may include character recognition capabilities for conversion of text-images to text. EMRs can accept codified clinical results from external sources like laboratories, radiological reports, disease management programs, etc, or external medication details from pharmacies or PBMs.

- **Medication Orders** - EMRs can create fully documented prescription orders for the pharmacist and update the patient medication history. Systems provide medication lists from which the physician may sort by brand, generic name, or therapeutic class. Orders are checked for dosages in excess of recommended ranges (as the case might be with off-label use), or may offer a dosing calculator based on patient age, weight, etc. Orders may include over the counter drugs, vitamins, supplements, etc. Prescriptions may be sent directly to pharmacies electronically or via fax until e-prescribing technology reaches its full capability. Systems have the ability to communicate and obtain patient eligibility, prior authorizations, drug formulary, and patient co-pay information from PBMs. Additionally, they capture acknowledgments, inquiries, and fill / refill notifications from pharmacies. The samples dispensed are recorded in the patient's medication history, and prescribed drugs are associated to a diagnosis. These systems can generate alerts for follow-up lab tests for certain medications that are known to have certain effects (such as toxicity, for example). EMRs provide support for drug interaction prevention-utilizing databases, which are updated on a regular basis. The systems check and issue alerts for potential interactions between a prescribed medication and the current medication list of the patient, medication allergies and intolerances, drug-disease interaction, and patient age. They also warn about the known impact of the medication on test results, as well as medications that are noted as having been ineffective on the patient in the past.

- **Diagnostic Test Orders** - EMR systems generate and manage orders for diagnostics, laboratory testing and imaging studies. The tests are associated with the patient's problem or diagnosis. An active order list informs the physician of pending tests, while the system provides historical lists of tests by type or associated diagnosis. The system records the ordering provider information. The user has the ability to review orders and send them to a provider by fax or electronically. EMR systems provide results management capabilities in that they notify relevant providers for review with inbox messages or updates and alerts in to-do lists. The systems can route results for review, allow assignment of reviewer responsibilities to clinical personnel, link results to orders, allow for free-text annotation, and associate image documents with tests. Test results are indicated as normal or abnormal based on acceptable value ranges that are specific to the results.

- **Referrals** - EMRs can create patient referrals for further care with specialists, physical therapists, speech therapists, and nutritionists. Additionally, they can issue non medication and non-clinical orders.

- **Patient Instructions** - The systems provide patient access to educational material, either through internal or external sources or via instructions pertaining to medication, tests, and procedures.

- **Patient Health Record** - EMR systems provide functionality for creating patient summary reports, listing current problems, medications, allergies and reactions. Reports may include all or part of patient record. Depending on the purpose of the report, it may or may not include encrypted data for patient privacy.

- **Consents, Authorizations and Directives** - EMRs can store and display image documents chronologically, along with online forms related to consents and patient authorizations. In addition, they can record advance directives documents, such as living wills, durable power of attorney, "Do not Resuscitate" orders, etc.

- **Decision Support** - EMR systems provide access to and the ability to maintain standard care plans, protocol, and guideline documents for physician decision support. These are either internal and site-specific documents, or from an external source such as an organization, payer, etc., and may include clinical trial protocols. Providers consult these references in order to make decisions related to the patient's care.

- **Disease Management, Preventive Services and Wellness** - EMR systems provide functionality for establishing criteria for disease management, wellness, and preventive care based on patient demographics and clinical data, such as diagnoses and current medications. The criteria are derived from guidelines issued by payers, national organizations, or internal protocols. Systems issue alerts and reminders for services due based on these guidelines, and have the ability to document all disease management, wellness, and preventive care activities related to a patient.

- **Administrative** - EMR systems provide functionality for a number of administrative tasks, from patient appointment scheduling to data retention, availability and destruction, audit trailing, and HIPAA confidentiality enforcement.

The Institute of Medicine of the National Academy of Sciences report on "Key Capabilities of an Electronic Health Record System" provides a view on the scope of these systems. The scope describes in broad terms the expected functionality present in EMR systems. Additionally, the Certification Commission of Healthcare Information Technology (CCHIT) is the recognized certification agency for electronic health record systems.

Unlike claims data which is based on industry standard formats, EMR databases are not designed to conform to any specific standards. The above functionality is not translated to a standard set of data fields that may be used be used in EMR systems. Software vendors rely frequently on their engagement with physician practices for the design of their software systems.

SOAP Notes Software

SOAP notes software is an abbreviated form of an EMR system. It is a software module that focuses on a single area: patient charting. Patient charting is perhaps the most important activity of the physician's document of the patient's care. Because of the significance of this activity and because of the difficulty in implementing full EMR systems, physicians opt for simpler technology utilization via SOAP notes software.

SOAP charting is based on the Subjective-Objective-Assessment-Plan (S-O-A-P) method of patient charting that physicians usually follow to document a patient encounter. SOAP notes are written by physicians, physician assistants, and nurse practitioners. Medical assistants may input subjective and objective observations, but the assessment and plan are always written by the professional. The SOAP model has four parts:

- **SUBJECTIVE:** This section captures subjective observations as expressed by the patient or his/her representative. It typically includes the reason for the visit, as well as the patient's symptoms and complaints, such as pain, discomfort, dizziness, etc.

- **OBJECTIVE:** This section captures the objective observations. These include the measurable observations of diagnostic tests and vital signs, such as temperature, pulse, swelling, blood pressure, respiration, skin color, height, weight, etc.

- **ASSESSMENT:** The assessment is the diagnosis of the patient's condition. A patient may be diagnosed with more than one condition, and where a clear assessment cannot be made, this section may list a number of possible diagnoses.

- **PLAN:** The plan outlines a course of action for the patient's care, which may include laboratory, radiological tests, prescribed medications, medical procedures, patient referral to specialists, patient orders and directions, etc.

SOAP notes capture a vital part of the patient's record. However, when compared to the scope of EMR systems, SOAP notes are severely limited. Because there are no requirements of how much information to provide, SOAP notes may vary in comprehensiveness. In addition, system design may vary considerably, and the design may include structured and free-text data elements. SOAP software, in the long run, may prove to be inadequate as more physicians migrate to systems with full functionality. However, in the short run they are a viable choice for patient charting information and analysis.

Continuity of Care Record

The Continuity of Care Record (CCR) is a snapshot in time of a patient's healthcare record. It captures the most essential facts about a patient's health status and treatments, and it is particularly useful in provider-to-provider communications. A referring physician can summarize and transfer the patient's information to the referred physician, who in turn, using the information on the CCR is able to learn all of the relevant facts about the patient. The CCR is to be updated by the practitioner with the most recent information after each new healthcare encounter with the patient.

The CCR is an information content standard that defines the data elements to be communicated. It was developed by ASTM International, a standards development organization, with participation from the American Academy of Family Physicians, the American Medical Association, the American Academy of Pediatrics, the Massachusetts Medical Society, the Patient Safety Institute, and the Health Information Management Systems Society (HIMSS). The CCR consists of the following blocks of information:

- Provider Identification and last services
- Patient Identification
- Insurance/health plan information
- Advance Directives
- Patient Health Status
  - Condition
  - Diagnosis or Problems
  - Family history
  - Social history & health risk factors
  - Adverse reactions, allergies, etc.
  - Medications
  - Immunizations
  - Vital signs & physiological measurements
  - Laboratory results, imaging & observations
  - Procedures
- Care documentation
  - Encounter history – dates, purpose, physician, etc.
- Care recommendation
  - Planned/scheduled tests/procedures or regimens of care
- Practitioners

In the absence of a widespread communication capability for sharing patient information between sites of care, the CCR is fast becoming the preferred means of communication of the patient's medical information. The recognized importance of the CCR has led to the development of the CCR Acceleration Task Force, which includes providers, EMR vendors, Patient Health Record (PHR) vendors, telecommunication vendors, and others. It is designed to speed up the development of system functionality and adoption the CCR standard for exchanging health data.

One critical element of CCR for the purpose it was developed is its portability. The CCR needs to be easily transferable from care site to care site. A patient's CCR can be printed out and transported by a patient or other authorized person, stored on a transportable electronic device (such as memory stick or compact disc), sent by fax, or electronically via email. In a more structured electronic environment, the CCR can be transmitted as a standard HL7 message, or an XML message that may be integrated into an EMR system. Given the course of the technology, it is envisioned that the CCR may eventually be transmitted via widely used electronic devices such as cell phones, mp3 players, and other devices.

The significance of a standard like the CCR in a non-standard environment such as the EMR is that it presents an opportunity for at least partial consistency between systems. These systems can now comply with a minimum standard: the CCR. The benefits from this consistency often leads to the development of other standards, which eventually lead to even more consistency. Also, with the enhanced information transfer between sites, patient records are more complete and can be found in more places. Ultimately, all of the above aid the processes of data collection and database building.

From the data standpoint, as a standard, the CCR has the potential of being used as a data collection instrument, regardless of how optimal the field collection is. When data is input into an EMR system, it has the potential of populating new data elements in the system, thus, enhancing the patient record database. One drawback with this is that the CCR includes mandatory and optional data elements, with the physician having sole discretion on what optional items are included in the transfer. That leaves some opportunity for inconsistency with the population of the CCR data elements, and it may have an effect on database integrity.

The CCR is a positive development within the EMR scope. However, one must consider the larger issue of the industry converging towards the same point when it comes to the data elements captured and the coding of these data elements. The CCR standard gives direction and defines a common denominator of data elements for EMR systems. That common denominator may prove too narrow to meet certain data needs, but in the absence of a comprehensive standard, it is a very valuable starting point.

EMR System-Adopted Standards

Even though EMR systems are not based on standards that define data elements, EMR systems have adopted certain standards for data values. Both aim to accomplish different goals, and there is a clear distinction between them. Data field standards precisely define the number of fields, names, value types, sizes, position, and order of the fields. Independently, data value standards provide lists of acceptable values that can be populated in data fields. This serves a very important role in the exchange of data. Various parties can communicate by referring to the same thing through using the same name without any ambiguities. File layout standards may exist with or without the existence of data value standards, and vice versa.

Claims data conforms both to layout and value standards. The scope of the claims process is finite and, therefore, it is possible to define all of the necessary data elements and arrange them so that one may produce a layout standard. The process of providing care is infinitely complex, and as a result, it cannot be definitively described by a set of data fields, regardless of the extent of the field set. When that happens, it is usually the case that the database allows flexibility with the use of free text fields. Additionally, it makes use of multi-variable fields that can store varying types of information. In the case of multi-variable fields, a predefined value describes the variable itself, with a separate value used as the actual measure of the variable. For example, a value of "Body Temperature" may describe the variable measured while a value of "98" is the actual measurement.

EMR systems capture both descriptive and coded information and have adopted a number of industry standard code sets. These code sets represent values of single variables as in the case of the ICD-9, CPT, and NDC codes, or may be also used to describe variables as in the case of medical term standards. In this case, the variable may be described with a standard medical term. Below are some of the adopted standards.

- **ICD-9:** International Code of Disease, 9th edition
- **CPT:** Current Procedural Terminology
- **HCPCS:** HCFA Common Procedural Coding System
- **NDC:** National Drug Codes
- **SNOMED CT®: S**ystematized **No**menclature of **Med**icine Clinical Terms
- **MEDCIN®** clinical engine
- **LOINC®:** Logical Observation Identifiers Names and Codes
- **DSM-IV™:** Diagnostic and Statistical Manual of Mental Disorders
- **HL7:** Health Level Seven

- **XML:** A standard for communication interfaces

SNOMED CT is a code set that provides standard clinical terminology. It is used to describe a variety of things, including clinical findings, observations, procedures, substances, organisms, specimens, objects, events, situations, products, etc. It uses terms and descriptions for identification, hierarchies, and relationships that link and associate items, and attributes that clarify them. SNOMED CT was developed by merging the SNOMED Reference Terminology of the College of American Pathologists (CAP) and the Clinical Terms Version 3 (CTV3) of the National Health Service (NHS) of United Kingdom. The terminology is used in computerized applications for capturing, aggregating, and communicating health data. SNOMED coding has applications in electronic medical records, medical research studies, clinical trials, disease surveillance, etc.

MEDCIN is a clinical vocabulary of 270,000 data elements, covering symptoms, history, physical examination, tests, diagnoses and therapy. It is used to create and maintain electronic documentation for patient encounters. MEDCIN is a product of Medicomp Systems, Inc, and evolved from their collaboration with physicians on staff from Cornell, Harvard, Johns Hopkins, and other medical centers. MEDCIN can be cross-mapped to ICD-9, CPT-4, HCPCS, LOINC, and DSM-IV code sets.

Even though SNOMED and MEDCIN appear to have competing scopes, SNOMED, as a reference terminology, is used to codify text data after it has been captured by an EMR system. SNOMED was not intended to be used at the point of care for entering information into the EMR system. MEDCIN, on the other hand, features medical terminology used for direct input into an EMR system. MEDCIN terms are fully mapped to the SNOMED terminology database, allowing for interoperability between the two languages. SNOMED, however, cannot map its clinical database to MEDCIN.

LOINC® is a standard clinical terminology for laboratory test orders and results. It is used for the electronic exchange and gathering of clinical results between health care facilities, laboratories, laboratory testing devices, and public health authorities. LOINC was developed and is maintained by the Regenstrief Institute.

DSM-IV, the Diagnostic and Statistical Manual of Mental Disorders, is the standard used by mental health professionals to classify mental disorders. It consists of three major components: the diagnostic classification, the diagnostic criteria sets, and the descriptive text. The diagnostic classification is the list of the mental disorders. Diagnostic classifications are mapped to ICD-9 diagnosis codes. The diagnostic criteria are a set of criteria that indicate the symptoms that must or must not be present in order for the patient to qualify for a diagnosis. The descriptive text is a systematic description of the disorder. The DSM is published by the American Psychiatric Association.

The HL7 is an electronic messaging standard for formatting and communicating electronic health data. It is a HIPAA adopted standard. It is used in the exchange of information between hospitals, practices, labs, imaging centers, remote home devices, etc. HL7, for example can be used to send a lab order request to a laboratory or diagnostic center and receive the results back. The HL7 does not specify what content is to be transmitted, but rather how the content will be structured and formatted. By contrast, the CCR is a standard specifying clinical content. Similar to HL7, the XML is a standard formatting language, though it is not specific to healthcare. Both the CCR and HL7 messages use XML as their architectural backbone.

The SNOMED, MEDCIN, LOINC, and DSM-IV code sets are not used in claims data because the clinical data in claims is limited to diagnosis, procedure, and drug use; the ICD-9, CPT, HCPCS, and NDC code sets are sufficient for such data. However, the use of these new code sets in patient data is extremely important in the electronic communication of data. A lack of coding standards means that one must use full text descriptions instead, which leaves a tremendous problem of misspelling and resolving ambiguous entries, thereby burdening the process. Codified data promotes system interoperability, as one system is able to recognize the terms of another.

Opportunities of EMR Data

How does EMR data present new opportunities? Considering the fact that claims data is broadly available and serves as a cornerstone of patient data today, one must start by examining the unmet needs of patient data. This includes examining existing applications enhanced with the use of EMR data, as well as new applications that were not previously possible with claims data.

The first opportunity is presented from the broad access to detailed evidence-based information. The wealth of medical information in EMR systems will more than likely encroach into the realm of primary market research. Traditionally, the healthcare industry relied partly on secondary data and partly on primary market research for answers to questions. With EMR data, more focus is shifted further to the objectivity of the patient data and away from subjective survey input. The reason for this is clear: the researcher will no longer have to rely on what the physician said, but what the physician did. Their data becomes their own testimony. During an interview, the physician may be questioned about their practicing habits. Typical questions like "how often," "what do you do in the case of," "how many times," etc., put the physician in the odd position to draw answers from memory with practically no chance of giving an accurate response. These and other questions with a retrospective focus are better answered with precise calculations that come with the usage of actual data. Studies based on secondary data can use a large number of physicians as subjects as opposed to the limited number of physicians normally used in primary market research studies. This also eliminates the possibility of emotions and bias interfering with a study.

The key strength of claims data is its breadth of scope in covering drug utilization, clinical, and charge information. However, the clinical data in the claims is the weak link. EMR clinical data is systematic and comprehensive. It captures essential details of the patient's treatment and provides the reasoning behind the physician's decisions. The physician's notes, vital signs data, and physiological measurements are all usable data for this purpose. Claims data provides limited visibility to lab data from the reimbursement standpoint. For example, evidence that a test was performed is visible, but the actual lab values are not. Lab values are a key component of EMR data. Together with vital signs, physiological measurements, and physician notes, they provide the evidence that helps to explain a physician's actions that cannot be seen through the claims data: for example, why certain procedures were performed, medications were changed, therapies terminated, new medication therapies initiated, etc.

One area where EMR data has a profound effect is in disease staging. Staging is by far more important to oncology than any other disease. Staging data is important to manufacturers for calculating business opportunity. Calculations are based on the drug's indicated line of therapy, the line of therapy-to-staging association, and the number of patients by disease stage. Although not explicitly stated in claims data, disease staging can in many cases be estimated by analyzing procedure and medication therapy data. Using empirical knowledge, analysts can associate surgical or radiological procedures, drug therapies, drug regimens, and therapy start data with disease stages. This indirect method has been a compromise, however: EMR data offers a more precise way to determine staging. EMR systems have the ability to explicitly capture the stage of the disease. For oncology, staging can also be captured indirectly through the tumor-node-metastasis (TNM) field values, discussed in more detail in a later section.

EMR data also provides new perspectives in drug dosing in both the retail and outpatient settings. EMR data captures the actual dosing schedules that are absent in pharmacy claims data. Claims data frequently allows analysts to calculate the average daily dosage from the days of therapy and quantity dispensed, but does not indicate the dosing frequency. In the physician's office, EMR data shows the exact dose administered. By contrast, claims based J-code drug data is assumed to be dosed at the amount represented by the J-code and the number of units. The data also highlights differences between suggested dosing, in relation to weight and body mass, and the actual dosing.

EMR data provides a new and unique perspective into prescription data, which is of the utmost importance to the manufacturer. Because the great majority of drug samples are dispensed by the physician, and therefore not captured in script data, the importance of samples is hardly weighed in any data analysis. Samples are given by physicians for a trial period at the beginning of a therapy. Depending on the effect of the drug samples on the patient, the physician determines the continuation of the therapy on the drug given or an alternative. Sample dispensing is not in the calculated results of therapy start and drug switching studies. These studies assume that the patient's first use of a drug in any class is the first pharmacy-dispensed prescription. Furthermore, a therapy switch is the change from the pharmacy-dispensed drug to another pharmacy-dispensed drug in the class.

EMR data may provide other prescribing perspectives as well. Barring the limited e-prescribing today, it can reconcile written and dispensed prescriptions. EMR systems have the capability of capturing physician-written scripts and the dispensing status of the scripts with pharmacy updates through e-prescribing, from which they may calculate the ratio of filled-to-written scripts. Prescription data from claims does capture pharmacy substitutions, but there is simply no way to determine the number of prescriptions written, but not filled. That number provides a new outlook on the treated versus untreated patient population, with a measure of refused treatment. Unfilled prescriptions are a missed opportunity for manufacturers, and a problem they could deal with by using patient education and co-pay assistance programs.

Another advantage of EMR clinical data is the sequencing and timing of events. EMR systems offer functionality to date and time-stamp events such as orders, dispensing, administration, testing, etc. This information is important when analyzing clinical data to precisely determine how the patient's care was delivered. Without the ability to sequence events, one cannot determine the cause of action or the responses to the events; for example, in determining if a medication is an add-on therapy or a substitution for a therapy.

Allergy, adverse reaction data, test results, and physician notes captured in EMR data all have the potential to explain the reasons behind drug switching. Claims data captures drug switching, but cannot explain the reasons. Manufacturers have to commission primary studies in order to understand drug switching. EMR data provides an alternative method by using factual data.

The Future of EMR Systems & Data

With only a fraction of the physician's offices using EMR systems in 2007, it will take a few more years before the technical environment and the physician's mindset are at a point that enables the market to reach critical mass. Today's EMR data comes mostly from specific specialties. Rightly so, because that is where the system installation base lies, and where data is needed most.

There is no question that the physician's practice will widely adopt the software in the future. This is a certainty because of a few reasons. The government is backing the change for economic reasons, as it anticipates high savings; this is shown through initiatives for system acceptance such as DOQ-IT, the efforts for the development of standards, HIPAA, etc. Payers have an interest here as well, again with economic reasons mostly in mind. Payers are looking for the savings that from better coordination of care, less duplication, and fewer unnecessary services.

But for this effort to succeed the providers must want it—providers do want it, because it enables them to provide better care to their patients and allows them to run their business more effectively. One important feature of the EMR data is in decision support with diagnosis and treatment. Making the right diagnosis through the appropriate testing, performing the right procedures, dispensing the right medication, and preventing side effects is not only the basis of good care, but it prevents malpractice lawsuits. Additionally, disease management and periodic preventive care is better managed by using computer technology with alerts, prompts, and messaging.

Usable EMR data is not going to happen simply because government, payers, and providers want to see that EMR technology succeeds. Successful implementation could serve the interests of these stakeholders without necessarily resulting in good data for the manufacturer. For that to happen, manufacturers and data vendors must agree on what is good data, and how it best serves research projects. In turn, vendors must distill that information to determine the required data elements, design the proper databases, and contract additional sources for the right data. Data vendors ought to be able to influence system designers and data aggregators to produce usable data. While claims databases in the market today are very similar, vendors implementing innovating solutions with EMR databases will be able to differentiate themselves.

Then comes the task of solving some technical problems. The first deals with the codification of free-text information. With many systems being text-based and data analysis requiring coded values, vendors may have to deal with extensive text-to-code conversions in order to produce usable databases. The second deals with the integration of disparate data sources. We must not lose sight of the fact that the integration of claims data from multiple suppliers is easy only because claims are based on data element and coding standards. Not only is it easy with claims data to define one's data inputs, but it is also easy to identify the same fields. EMR data is based partly on coding standards, but not on data element standards. Even though desired metrics are likely to be captured by the various EMR systems, the

127

cross-walking of the data elements is something the vendors will have to resolve. Also troubling is the fact that EMR data is not uniform across specialties; to document care for certain specialty conditions, it requires additional data elements. Therefore, EMR data solutions must deal effectively with exceptions. A third technical issue has to do with data encryption. Data encryption in claims is as simple as determining the data columns to encrypt. In EMR data, the patient information is embedded and repeated in free-text frequently. Removing references to the patient's identity will likely prove challenging.

Of course, the role of physician cannot be overlooked here. Aside from the fact that the success of EMR data hinges on a broad system installation base, physician compliance with data input is the second most critical issue. The data fields must be populated for good data to occur. The physician must be willing to record and sufficiently code the patient encounter. EMR software designers seem to realize this fact now, and newer, more sophisticated system designs make the task easier and faster for the physician to document. Also, newer and future generations of physicians will probably fare better in terms of working with computer systems.

There are three possible key scenarios that could unfold in the evolution of the EMR data. The first is that EMR data remains a limited application dataset for a small number of therapeutic areas, much like its present state. This scenario does not hold much incremental potential for any stakeholder. Under a second scenario, EMR data reaches its full potential as the result of successful implementation and physician compliance with data input. This would be the ultimate scenario, and one that would put EMR in direct competition with claims data. However, at best this would occur in the distant future. The third scenario, which falls short of the second but complements the first, is that full scale implementation databases are constructed from rather small, specialty-stratified panels of incentivized physicians. This concept is used in survey databases today, and could even be an interim solution to the second scenario. An EMR database with the aforementioned capabilities, even in a small scale, would be a tremendous market research resource.

EMR vs. Claims Data

EMR data, unquestionably, has great future potential. The reality, however, is that today's databases are very limited. Not only do they focus on few specialties, mainly oncology, but they are also limited to certain data elements. Driven by manufacturer's data needs, often revolving around drug dosing and disease staging, vendors have designed early products to address just that. We will qualify these databases as EMR products, even though the definition leaves room for debate. Every available data element has potential for providing a new perspective when analyzed, and even though EMR data has a more profound impact on certain specialties, every specialty could reap some benefits from data analysis. With that in mind, true EMR data will have to come a very long way to contend for first place against claims data.

Claims data, on the other hand, is now in a mature state by virtue of how extensive the use of electronic claims is today and the fact that claims are based entirely on predefined standards. Even with claims data, however, there is opportunity for new applications. While initially the industry focused on the obvious, analysis of the data is becoming more sophisticated, with analysts taking a harder look at the data. There are still unexplored data elements in claims data whose analytical value has not been determined yet, and applications such as field compensation are but a striking distance away, given the universe coverage. As it stands today, claims data is the key patient data type. Not only does it cover drug utilization more comprehensively, it provides great insights into clinical care and offers exclusive perspectives into the financial aspects of the healthcare industry. And while with time, EMR data has the potential of outperforming claims with richer drug and clinical data, the financial data is not even in its scope.

But this is not really about making a choice between one and the other. The ultimate data solution is based on integrated data from both claims and EMR, as well as other data sources. However, building this integrated solution requires an important decision to be made first. This solution is built from smaller building blocks, and following the fundamental principles of building, you must decide what block to set as the foundation. Such principles dictate that the most substantial block is set down first. A solution where the fundamental building block is claims data will look different than a solution where EMR is used as the foundation. With claims as the key data type, EMR assumes the backup role of filling in for the weaknesses of claims clinical data. Examples of that today include the lab values data integrated into claims and the oncology dosing and staging data. With EMR and its robust clinical data as the key data type, claims assume the role of supplying the charge data, with its role potentially limited to that.

Today, setting the EMR block down first is not an option because EMR databases lack both breadth and depth. The question is this: will it in the future? The answer to that is hard to predict, although it is clear what it depends on. It will take the very successful implementation of EMR technology for that happen, and the odds of that are hard to calculate. Successful implementation will not only be measured simply in terms of the size of the installed user base, but more importantly, in the adherence to data input requirements and the proliferation of peer-to-peer and partner-to-partner data exchanges. Failure of physicians to document encounters thoroughly will compromise the integrity of the data. Also, limited data exchanges will not solve the problem seen in most claims databases of partial patient records. At least on paper, EMR technology holds the promise of better integration of the patient's history from multiple sources.

Today, visualizing ultimate solution is a puzzle, with the role of claims data being the most crucial element, as it provides the foundation for drug, clinical, and charge data for all indications. The hospital drug utilization limitation of claims data is dealt with charge master-level data. Finally, EMR and survey databases, when possible, provide additional insights for certain specialties.

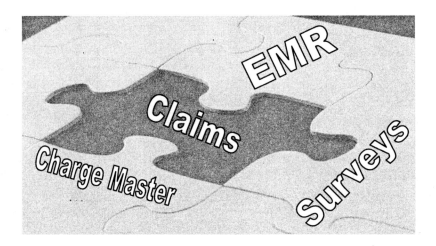

Figure 11: *Patient data current scenario*

If the adoption of EMR technology was very successful, EMR would have a chance of becoming the puzzle's center piece. In that scenario, charge data would be supplemented from claims, charge master-level data would not be necessary because it would be embedded in the EMR data, and survey databases would become obsolete.

Chapter 5
Applications

What sets patient data apart from other data types is the range of applications that the data is applicable for. A key first step in dealing with these applications is selecting the appropriate set of data for the study. Considering the different data offerings in the market and the limitations of these products, that means selecting a database that best fits the particular application. With other data products, manufacturers typically commit to a data offering from a particular vendor, and for the shake of consistency and cost considerations, would use the product for all of the projects. With patient data applications, manufacturers must maintain relationships with multiple vendors simply because a single vendor's products cannot address all of the company's needs. Selecting the right patient database for the project requires a good understanding of the data offerings.

The database characteristics to look for when selecting a product for a project are timeliness, completeness, patient type representation, payer type representation, attribute limitations, and data integration. The timeliness of the data is a relative concept and has to do with the frequency of database updates and the time lag of the reported period. For pharmacy claims, data timeliness can be measured in days and charge master-level data in weeks. For hospital claims, on the other hand, timeliness is measured in months because of the time it takes to adjudicate the majority of a hospital's claims. Some databases are not published until all of the claims for a reporting period are processed and paid. This is usually several months past the reporting period. Other databases only track the paid claims up to the most reporting period, even though other claims from the same period are still pending. Databases that use submitted claims will be timelier than databases using paid claims.

A key difference between databases is the type of patient covered. All databases cover the managed care patient, for example. However, the cash paying patient is visible in fewer databases. Similarly, the payer is important in many studies, and databases vary on the basis of payer types covered. Some databases make restrictive use of certain data elements. Physician visibility, for example, may be limited to specialty, and payer visibility to the plan type. In general, some databases are more inclusive than others.

Databases vary in their ability to integrate patient records from different sources. Closed-panel databases, although limited in other ways, are tightly integrated databases with more complete patient profiles. Open-panel databases use sophisticated patient matching algorithms to achieve a good level of data integration, but their strengths usually lie elsewhere. The complete perspective of the patient captured in closed-panel databases is more important to some applications, such as in outcomes and economic studies.

Then, there are the unique perspectives of databases. The payer actions observed through claims switch-sourced data are unique to that source. Other payer perspectives like patient enrollment, eligibility, benefit design, demographics, employer perspectives, and productivity measures are unique to some databases. The sample size is a very important determinant for the study that must be weighed against other criteria, but it is also a tricky one only because it can be misunderstood. Data vendors often boast of the value of their databases using statistics like the cumulative number of patients, years of data history, number of claims, etc. In reality, the only sample size that matters is what is left after all of the study criteria have been applied and the qualified records have been reduced to the minimum. A large database may still produce a suboptimal sample size to sufficiently address the business questions in a study.

There are several reasons why a study cannot be qualified on the size of the entire database. For the purpose of defining the most appropriate patient sample, the first step is to identify the patients who truly have the disease of interest. Most chronic diseases require the presence of two claims during the time period with the ICD-9 code for the disease in order to eliminate patients who don't actually have the disease, but may have a single claim with the diagnosis code of interest. In addition, patient inclusion in the sample may require the presence of specific CPT-4 codes, drug codes, or diagnosis codes associated with related comorbidities. These patients are further reduced to those that meet minimum requirements of months of history or the relative timing of the history. This is the result of patients becoming visible in the database at different times, either because they just enrolled in a plan, changed employer, provider, or pharmacy, or if they chose a new business partner, etc. Further study-specific requirements will reduce the sample even more. Figure 12 demonstrates an example of qualified patients for a study by number of years of history in the database.

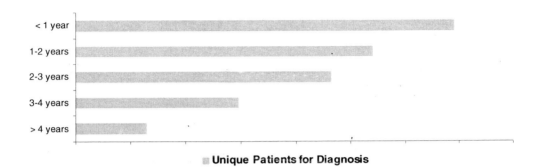

Figure 12: *Patients by length of data history – Courtesy of IMS Health*

The most critical part of a study is the definition of the business rules. This is a step that requires the very close cooperation of the data vendor and the client. Vendors may have their own standard methodology and definitions for a given application. However, clients often choose to modify certain rules or parameters in the study. Other data types are more straightforward, with fewer rules that are already embedded in the data. Patient data is unique in that respect, and therefore is highly customizable. It resembles more of a market research project than it does a data project. Defining and applying business rules are two sets of unique skills required for dealing with patient data.

Currently, vendors maintain the balance of power on their side where skills and knowledge are concerned, and most of the patient data studies are executed by them. Alternatively and less frequently, clients make use of their option to take raw data in house, applying their rules and producing their own reports. By comparison, working with patient data is many times more complex than dealing with sales data or prescription data: two typical applications that manufacturers deal with. In addition, patient data volume is overwhelmingly larger than any of the two. Then, there is the middle-of-the-road approach where the vendor stages the data in a data mart for direct access by the client in a semi-automated fashion, with query capabilities and many of the rules built into the system.

The flexibility of raw data to run an endless number of studies is very appealing until the realities of dealing with the data settle in. There is no easy way to determine if a company is up to the task, other than to make a quick assessment of how well they fare with the smaller, infinitely less complex sales and prescription applications. The reality is that even these applications are challenging for many.

The following section discusses a number of typical patient data applications, grouped into four different categories: treatment and utilization patterns, brand performance, epidemiology, and pharmacoeconomics.

Treatment and Utilization Patterns

Treatment and Utilization pattern applications focus on the different therapy modes for particular diseases, with the center of attention placed on the drug therapies in order to identify characteristics related to the use of the drugs. These studies also examine the role of the physician from the point of the patient's diagnosis to the patient referral and treatment.

Therapy Progression: This application analyzes the typical patterns of disease treatment, including drug, surgery, radiology, and other procedures from the first diagnosis to the later stages of the disease. It also studies the patient's length of therapies and the time it takes for the patient to advance between therapies.

The diagnosis of a disease does not automatically imply advanced therapy with the use of prescription drugs or procedures, but it may involve the use of an over-the-counter medication, or even the use of simple remedies for the relief of the symptoms, such as topical massage, soaking, liquid diets, etc. If there are preventive therapies, the physician will likely prescribe them. However, as the disease progresses, the patient may be put on different drug therapies, starting with low doses of milder drugs to progressively larger doses or stronger, potentially more toxic and more effective drug therapies. For some diseases, applicable therapies may include radiology, surgery, or other less-invasive procedures.

The order by which these therapies are administered is important, and the analysis of the data aims to identify the sequences. This is important for the drug manufacturer because not only might their drug may not be applicable as a therapy until a certain stage of the disease, but also because drug therapies often compete with non-drug therapies. Data analysis creates a map of the progression, creates a decision tree of the therapies, and helps the manufacturer determine the percent of the patient population that will reach the target range of their drug. Understanding this path allows manufacturers to better position their drugs against competing therapies. Figure 13 demonstrates the treatment path for patients with *Product A* as their first line of therapy.

The analysis further identifies therapy differences among practitioners. Age and sex cohort analysis is also important, as younger patients can sometimes better tolerate certain treatments and may be treated more aggressively; older patients with greater sensitivity to side effects and adverse reactions may be treated more conservatively.

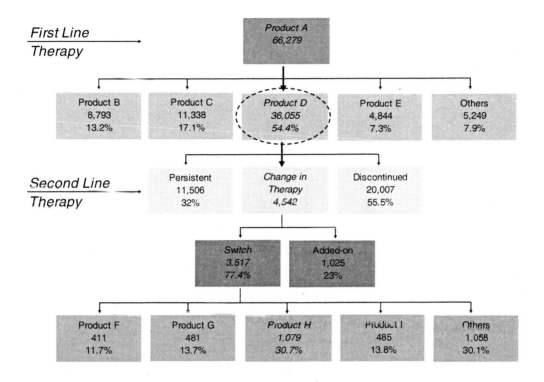

Figure 13: *Therapy progression — Courtesy of SDI, Inc.*

Another relevant aspect of the pattern of care is the place of therapy. For non-drug therapies, that includes identifying where the procedures are performed, be they inpatient, outpatient, in physician office settings, or at other ancillary facilities. For drug therapies, the process involves identifying whether the drugs are self-administered or administered at a physician's office, infusion center, hospital, etc. In addition, the analysis attempts to identify the frequency of office visits, which are often tied to the prescription length.

Many of the studies focus on retail claims in order to identify the first and subsequent lines of therapy. A comprehensive analysis includes both medical and pharmacy claims analyses to identify the drug and non-drug therapies. When a market includes retail and injectable or infusion drugs, drug therapy analysis would also require the use of medical claims for clinical and hospital utilization. For inpatient hospital drug utilization, charge master-level data is necessary to identify the drugs used.

Therapy progression studies require a cohort of patients with an initial diagnosis and enough data history to capture the progression from one therapy to another. These studies can be performed with either open or closed-panel databases. For drug therapy progression analysis, the open-panel databases provide large pharmacy claims data samples. For drug and medical therapy progression analysis, the sample size for qualifying patients is reduced considerably, as not every patient with pharmacy claims will have medical claims in the database. Alternatively, closed-panel databases are good at integrating drug and medical claims, and they include all of the patient's therapies. The applicable drug therapies for the study are defined by the classes of drugs indicated for the treatment of the disease. The use of diagnosis codes from medical claims may be necessary to distinguish between multiple drug indications in some studies. Procedures are qualified by their ICD-9 or HCPCS codes.

Claims data analysis provides an adequate view of the paths of therapy, but not a comprehensive one. Claims data cannot identify therapies beyond prescription drugs or procedures, such as OTC drugs, drug samples, and other remedies. These patients are grouped in the untreated category, and their time from initial diagnosis to treatment is miscalculated. This leaves an opportunity for future EMR data to provide a more accurate perspective.

Drug Dosing & Titration:
Drug dosing applications analyze the average daily consumption of a drug and produce a distribution of dosages by patient population. Dosing is important to manufacturers from both the outcome and economic standpoints: first, because inappropriate dosing does not produce the optimal medical outcomes, and second, to maximize revenue.

For retail drugs, dosing is calculated by dividing the quantity dispensed by the days of therapy. Drugs may be dosed one or more times every day or every n^{th} day. However, lack of information on the claim does not allow for precise calculations at that level. Therefore, analysis is limited to an assumed daily average. The calculations are easy to perform for certain drugs like pills, where the number of pills is divided by the number of days. For other products like creams, sprays, ointments and injectables, for which the number of days of therapy is often not provided, the average daily consumption can be calculated by using the number of doses per container divided by the average days between refills in lieu of the days of therapy. Business rules can be added to account for non-compliant patients.

For physician's office and hospital outpatient drug administration, dosing is calculated from claims data based on the J-Code of the administered drug. J-Codes are set for reimbursing a specific amount of a drug, i.e. 10mg. Thus, the administered dose is equal to the J-Code amount times the number of units administered. Physician's office and hospital outpatient drug procedures are billed individually, and professional claims capture the administration intervals between days (but exclude intra-day administrations). Inpatient hospital drug utilization data is available only in the hospital's charge master-level data and captures the product and quantity dispensed with the date of administration. The charge master-level data also captures outpatient hospital drug utilization.

Titration is the process of determining the right dosing of a drug for a patient. The approved dosing of a drug is the dosing that would have a therapeutic benefit to the majority of patients. The appropriate dosing for a specific patient is a function of one or more factors, including the patient's test results, body mass, weight, age, etc. Physicians often use various titration methods to arrive at the patient's proper dosing. Titration where an immediate effect is desired or acute conditions starts with higher doses and gradually reduces the dose to the desired or optimal level. When no immediate response is required, physicians may titrate with lower doses and gradually increase until the desired results have been achieved.

Manufacturers initiate titration data analysis for the purpose of identifying trends for their product and competing products. They also use titration analysis to identify low titrating physicians. Physicians may then be targeted to increase dosing and maximize the therapeutic benefit of the drug, and by extension, the revenue of the drug company. The study involves analysis of a cohort of patients by using pharmacy claims for a period of time and observing the dosing variations in a patient's history. Titration studies may also include plan data for plan influence analysis. The analysis often focuses on cross-product titration differences for switched patients. Manufacturers sometimes use titration analysis to defend against switching when switching results in an increased cost of therapy due to higher titration.

Dosing analysis ideally should take into consideration the patient's test results, body mass, weight, age, etc. Presently, however, only data for certain lab results, usually from independent labs, is available for analysis, and only for a limited number of patients. As a result, the scope of the dosing analysis is rather limited; often, further primary market research is needed. EMR data has the opportunity to change that in the future, as it offers better capture of test results and patient physiometric data. In addition, it could provide precise dosing information with daily frequencies. Early partial EMR data for specialties like oncology provide dosing by drug and drug regimen.

Mode of Drug Therapy: The mode of therapy analysis attempts to answer two key questions: how many drugs patients are on at the same time for the treatment of a disease, and what are the most common drug regimens? When a patient is treated using a single drug, the patient is said to be on mono-therapy. Often, patients respond better to treatments using more than one drug, and in that case, the patient is said to be on combination therapy. There may be multiple drug combinations used to treat a disease from the same or different classes of drugs within a therapeutic area.

Patients on multiple drugs for the treatment of the same disease are not necessarily on combination therapy unless they have been on the drugs concomitantly. A prescription for a new drug for a patient previously on mono-therapy does not automatically qualify as concomitant therapy because the patient may have filled one prescription and subsequently switched to another drug during the reporting period. Prescriptions filled on the same day are most likely intended for combination therapy, but not all concomitant use prescriptions are filled on the same day. A physician may have seen the patient and prescribed a new medication "out of cycle" with the original drug. The uncertainty regarding overlapping days of therapy is resolved by looking forward to subsequent data periods to assure that both prescriptions were re-filled. Otherwise, a therapeutic substitution is assumed.

The study must define and limit the drugs that would be considered concomitant for the treatment of a disease to distinguish them from drugs used for non-related conditions and drugs that are always a switch, such as switching from one proton pump inhibitor to another. Pharmacy claims data is usually sufficient for these studies when the market involves retail drugs only and multiple indications do not interfere with the analysis. Medical claims data may be required in cases where the drug class includes non-retail drugs with limited pharmacy claims, and to resolve the ambiguity of multiple indications.

Sometimes, the analysis is extended to unrelated classes of drugs in order to study concomitant drug utilization for comorbid conditions. Using pharmacy claims, analysts are able to identify different classes of drugs used at the same time for the treatment of different diseases. Comorbidities are conditions that exist at the same time with another disease. A comorbidity study focuses on the frequently occurring conditions with the disease of interest. Concomitant drug utilization due to comorbidities is determined by the presence of pharmacy claims for drug classes known to treat the comorbid diseases. A better approach uses medical claims to identify patients with certain diagnoses for comorbid conditions and studies the pharmacy claims for the same period of time for concomitant drug utilization. Comorbidity analysis is important for manufacturers when the existence of a condition inhibits the use of their drugs due to drug interactions, or when there is a need to explore potential opportunities for additional labeling indications.

Both open and closed-panel databases are suitable for these applications. For retail drug studies, open-panel databases provide large pharmacy samples, while closed-panel databases offer some advantages by including non-retail drugs, multi-indicated drugs, and diagnoses.

Referral Pattern Analysis: This analysis tries to identify how the patient is referred for care within the healthcare system between physician specialties and between facility types. It is a fact that the majority of diagnoses are made within physician practices and by the primary care physicians (PCPs). The reason is that managed care encourages the use of PCPs and requires a referral before a patient can see a specialist. PCPs do not treat every condition of every patient, especially when the condition is outside their specialization or when the disease is in more advanced stages, thus, referrals are generated in these cases. Another reason is that the patient seeks the advice of a PCP because they cannot self-diagnose and seek care directly from the right specialist. As more complex care is required, the patient may be referred from the practice to a clinic, hospital, rehabilitation center, long term care, etc.

Referral analysis is important for the manufacturer because of potential treatment differences between PCPs and specialists, as well as the settings of care. Specialists often switch the patient's drug therapy during the hand-off of the patient to their standard protocol. Manufacturers prefer the referrals to specialists due to the smaller number of professionals involved in the disease treatment, thus giving the manufacturer more control over their targeting activities.

Specialty referral analysis through using pharmacy claims involves the identification of the prescribing physicians and their specialties from the patient's prescriptions. The disease is qualified by relevant drug classes. This works only when the diagnosing physician initially treats the patient before the patient is referred to the specialist. Otherwise, medical claims are required to identify the diagnosing physician. Medical claims analysis is also required when non-retail drugs and drugs with multiple indications are involved. The analysis attempts to identify multiple physician specialties for the same patient and the same diagnosis.

Referral pattern analysis usually validates intelligence gathered by the sales force, but the study may have an additional benefit: a list of physicians for targeting purposes. Physicians may be segmented by their role and by volume. Certain primary care physicians refer many patients to a specialist but never see the patient again, as the specialist "keeps" the patient. However, certain specialists will treat the patient for a period of time and send the patient back to the PCP for continued and maintenance of medication treatment.

Referral analysis can be performed with open or closed-panel claims databases. Closed panel databases are particularly suited for specialty level analysis because they capture all of the patient's treating physicians and places of care. However, for physician-level analysis and to obtain a target list of physicians, only open-panel databases are likely to provide the identity of the physician and a sizable pharmacy claims sample.

Claims data does not support analysis that would identify the physician's determining factors to treat or refer because it lacks circumstantial data, such as disease severity and symptoms, test results, etc. These are data elements present in EMR systems, which analysts may be able to mine in the future.

Drug Use by Indication:

Determining the drug's sales by the indication is very important for manufacturers for two main reasons. First, there is considerable investment in clinical studies to develop and maintain a drug for an indication, and manufacturers need to be able to measure the drug's performance in the indication for ROI analysis. Second, the product, most likely, is supported with some level of sales and marketing for each indication, and manufacturers need to optimize their resource allocation based on potential. In addition, they must forecast sales and create the right incentives for the promotion of the indication. In targeting, for example, assigning the accounts to the right sales force is critical, or the wrong messages will be delivered to accounts.

The analysis provides the added benefit of identifying and monitoring off-label use of a drug, where applicable. Increased off-label use represents a risk for the manufacturer when a lot of product utilization is tied to an unapproved indication, and at the same time it presents an opportunity to pursue additional clinical studies in order to support broader labeling claims that could enable targeting of specific subpopulations. From the standpoint of safety, manufacturers can evaluate whether the drug is being misused in at-risk segments of the disease population.

Legacy sales and prescription data do not capture the patient diagnosis and do not offer any precise way of determining the indication for the products used in clinics and hospitals, or those that are dispensed from pharmacies. The specialty of the prescribing physician or the facility and the indicated strength of the product are used, where applicable, to approximate their use by disease category. For retail drugs, it is generally assumed that the indication of the dispensed drug is the indication closest to the specialty of the dispensing physician. Oncologist-written prescriptions are intended for oncological indications, and cardiologist-written prescriptions are intended for cardiological indications. For non-retail drugs, the general specialty classification of the clinic is used to determine the disease category of the product used. For hospitals without specialty classifications, one method used is based on related procedure data.

The problem with the specialty data is that for unclassified accounts or neutral physician specialties with no direct link to the disease category, the allocation is practically impossible. In those cases, empirical data pertaining to dosing and the method of administration for each indication is used to allocate the remaining data to disease categories. The indicated strength and form of a drug often would normally be used by themselves, or in combination with the specialty, specifically for that purpose. For example, if the high-dose, injectable form of the drug is used in oncology while the low-strength oral form is used in rheumatology, the associated data for these forms and strengths can be allocated to the applicable disease categories. Despite all of that, however, if a product has multiple indications within a disease category, i.e. breast and lung cancer within oncology, these methods are absolutely ineffective in determining the right indication.

Patient data offers the only precise method of determining drug utilization by indication by using the patient's diagnosis. For retail drugs, that is done by matching pharmacy claims data for a drug to professional and hospital claims data by using the patient ID and identifying the diagnoses. The analysis can be performed at the national level if the intent is to split revenues by indication, which is done by calculating the ratio of the normalized dispensed quantities for each diagnosis. Figure 14 demonstrates the use of *Brand-x* by diagnoses listed along the X axis.

If the intent is to use the data in a targeting application, the analysis must be done at the physician's specialty level to determine the specialty's influence on an indication. Each specialty's percent contribution can be calculated either at the brand, or for more precision, at the form and strength level. Physician specialties can be targeted accordingly using the results of the analysis.

For physician's office and clinic-administered drugs, the use by indication can be determined by matching diagnoses to the J-Coded drugs through using professional claims data to calculate the percentages of contribution of each indication for the segment as a whole. For a hospital's drugs, use by indication can be determined by using charge master-level data and matching drugs to diagnoses. For certain drugs that share the same J-Code or are referenced often using their generic name, the analysis is done at the molecular level, but it cannot be applied to the brand.

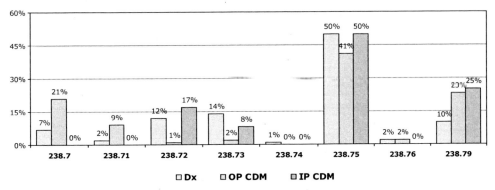

Figure 14: *Brand-x drug use by indication – Courtesy of SDI, Inc.*

Drug utilization by indication analysis should be repeated on a periodic basis, at least annually, because market dynamics may shift the balance between indications. Analysis at a level below national for targeting purposes is possible. However, the universe of covered accounts in claims databases is limited to a subset of accounts and the analysis would yield incomplete results. Physician-level analysis is frequently sub-optimal because not all physicians from the pharmacy claims can be matched to physicians from the professional claims. Similarly, only a fraction of physician's practices and hospitals would be visible in the claims data.

All database types are suitable for national and specialty-level drug utilization by indication analysis. For sub-national-level analysis, closed-panel databases would provide a broader coverage of providers but may limit the identification of the provider.

Treatment Adherence: Adherence measures the patient's commitment to their therapies and has two main components: persistence and compliance. Adherence applies to chronic therapies and therapies that extend over a few prescription fill periods. The concept is applicable also to acute conditions with a single prescription fill, as the patient still has to self-medicate regularly and for the entire prescribed period. However, the results are not measurable with patient data. Adherence applications are among the most important of all patient data applications, as the insights gained here have significant implications for patients, physicians, payers, and manufacturers.

Efficacious drugs deliver the maximum benefit to patients when they are prescribed at the right dose, taken at the right intervals, and taken without interruption for the prescribed period. Therefore, clinical outcomes depend significantly on the physician's correct assessment of the patient and the prescription of the right medication at the right dosing, as well as the patient's adherence to the prescription orders. Ultimately, drug therapies are measured by their outcomes and reflect on the physician and the drug.

For the manufacturer, aside from the fact that efficacy must be proven and that can be best demonstrated with proper medication, there is a financial stake as well. Manufacturers maximize their revenue when patients are both compliant and persistent with their therapies. Every missed dose, interruption in the therapy and premature termination of therapies represents a missed opportunity. Therefore, manufacturers must be fully aware of the degree of adherence and work with physicians, pharmacists, caregivers, managed care, and patients alike to ensure an optimal level of patient persistence and compliance.

For payers, there is a financial burden that goes along with a lack of adherence. Non-adherent patients are sicker and eventually consume more healthcare services. Adherence presents opportunities for the payer because it reduces disease progression, incidence of comorbid conditions and complications, and results in fewer hospital days, ER visits, primary care, and specialist visits.

- **Persistence:** Persistence measures the extent to which therapies are followed without significant interruptions from the time of initiation to termination. Interruption is defined as the grace period between the expected time of a prescription refill to the actual time of the fill. Assuming that the patient fills a thirty day prescription but refills after thirty five days, the patient has interrupted the therapy for five days but has not terminated the therapy. When the interruption exceeds an agreed length of time, the patient is deemed to have terminated their therapy. In many studies, a grace period of one month is usually considered. Terminated patients may restart their therapies, but the restarted period does not figure into the calculation of persistence.

  Persistence is measured either at the brand level or the treatment level. Patients are brand-persistent as long as they continue on their treatment with the given brand. Patients are treatment-persistent as long as they continue on the brand or switch to an alternative therapy without interruptions beyond the grace period.

  One approach to persistence is to identify a cohort of patients that initiated therapy during a specific time period, i.e. the previous month, quarter, etc. Therapy initiation is determined by examining a prior period of time to assure that the patient was not on the study drug during that period. The patient history must be visible in the database during this examination period. For subsequent reporting periods, typically months, the study classifies each patient in the cohort as:

    - **Persistent:** refilled prescription within grace period
    - **Switched:** still treated but on different drug
    - **Discontinued:** did not refill within grace period
    - **Restarted:** started therapy again after a down period

Based on the observations, a decay curve is constructed that shows the number of patients still on the drug (persistent) and the number of patients that dropped off (discontinued) the therapy with each subsequent month from the beginning of the study – see figure 15. For treatment persistence, the decay graph shows the number of patients still on therapy (persistent + switched) and the discontinued patients by month. The restarted patient count, although important to the manufacturer, bears no further relevance to the concept of persistence.

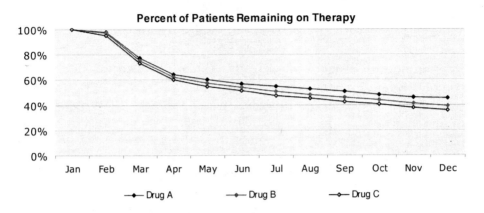

Figure 15: *Patient persistence – Courtesy of Wolters Kluwer*

The study usually picks new cohorts of initiated patients in subsequent periods and tracks them similarly over time. Using the Kaplan-Meier survival analysis technique or other similar techniques, analysts can forecast the time it will take for the cohort patients to drop off the therapy as shown in the graph above. Prospective persistence analysis is particularly suited for new brands or when there is a recent change in the marketplace that impacts the brand.

If the first cohort of patients is more recent, the longer it will take for the actual results to be measured. Persistence cohort studies may be done retrospectively, with historical data used to generate more immediate results. When that happens, because patients initiated their therapies at different time periods, their initiation periods (t0) and subsequent periods (t1, t2, …) are synchronized in order to measure the drop-off rates in reference to the initial period. The synchronization of time periods is referred to as time alignment.

- **Compliance:** Compliance measures the patient's adherence to the prescribed consumption of the drug. For a thirty-day prescription, for example, the patient is expected to consume the entire dispensed amount by the end of the thirty days. The patient is then expected to refill the prescription and begin consumption of the newly dispensed drug on the thirty-first day. When that happens, the patient is said to be 100% compliant. However, if the patient starts consumption of the newly dispensed drug beyond the thirty-first day, the patient is non-compliant.

The traditional method of measuring the rate of compliance uses the days of supply and quantity dispensed data elements in pharmacy claims. Compliance is defined as the ratio of days of supply for all prescriptions over a set time period to the total calendar days between the first and last script in the period. The total days of supply does not include the supply days of the last script.

Compliance = Days of Supply / Total Calendar Days

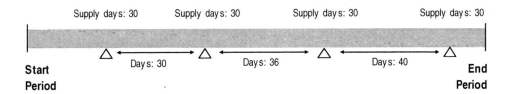

Figure 16: *Patient compliance*

In the above example, a patient has four fills within the time period of interest. Between the first and last script, the patient received 90 days of supply, which was consumed in a total of 106 days. Therefore, the patient was 85% compliant (90/106). Notice that the last 30 day supply is not included in the calculations because it applies to a subsequent period. Compliance rates are calculated for specific time periods, i.e. six or twelve-month periods for patients with at least two claims in the period, or for cohorts of patients over time with periodic recalculations.

Another method of calculating compliance is by using the Medication Possession Ratio (MPR). The MPR is calculated by dividing the quantity dispensed in the study period by the quantity of drug the patient needs for continuous use in the same time period. The quantity needed can be calculated by the average daily dose times the number of days in the period of interest.

Medication Possession Ratio = Qty. Dispensed / Qty. Needed

Patient adherence is affected by several factors. Some are as simple as the patient forgetting to take their medication in going about their daily routine. More frequent drug dosing, multiple drug regimens due to comorbidities, and age contribute to a lower adherence. Another reason is found in disease severity and drug side effects. Disease severity is often associated with higher doses of medications, which are in turn associated with higher levels of side effects. The patient's understanding of the disease is often a factor of non-adherence. Frequently, patients will stop their therapies because they feel better or because their tests reached a target range, only to relapse later. Experiencing pain and/or discomfort and the complexity of drug administration are other factors. The patient's price sensitivity is also a critical reason for non-adherence. Patients often defer re-filling their prescriptions due to economic reasons. This is significant enough that many times merits the analysis of persistence in conjunction with co-pay. Figure 17 demonstrates a refill analysis tracking the percent of refills at different time intervals from the time of the previous fill.

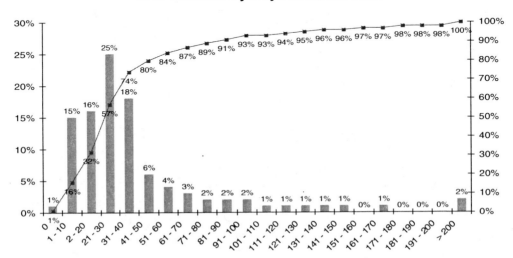

Figure 17: *Refill analysis – Source: Verispan LLC*

Adherence is increasingly used in patient segmentation by manufacturers who are interested in identifying non-adherent patient segments and targeting them with direct-to-patient programs and appropriate messaging. Similarly, in physician segmentation, manufacturers are looking for physicians whose patients exhibit low levels of adherence and target them appropriately with proper messaging, or by sharing information learned from more compliant physician groups. For physicians, improving adherence is clearly a matter of better disease management.

The concept of adherence is widely applicable to retail drugs and can be easily dealt with in pharmacy claims data. Adherence also applies to non-retail drugs as well, and can be dealt with in medical claims. For office-injectable and infusion drugs, the analysis focuses on administration patterns and the administration time intervals.

TIP: Certain drug therapies have irregular administration patterns. They may require a different initial dose and frequency than the on-going treatment. In these cases, a certain level of product knowledge may be required to interpret the results of the analysis.

For therapy-level adherence, analysts must be mindful of markets that include non-retail drugs as well. In that case, an integrated source of medical and pharmacy claims is required to capture product switches from retail to non-retail drugs, and vice versa. In rare occasions, and where a non-drug therapy is known to exist, a more comprehensive study may require the analysis of applicable procedure data in conjunction with drug usage.

Adherence calculations require accurate capture of every medication claim. Otherwise, compliance and medication possession rates can be understated. Missing scripts may cause patients to be deemed discontinued and dropped from the persistence cohorts. Closed-panel databases are most accurate for adherence applications in that respect. However, the latency of these databases makes them less suitable for prospective studies, adherence of new products, and products in dynamic markets. Open-panel databases, on the other hand, provide more real-time data and capture more retail claims, but they are potentially less accurate.

Brand Performance Applications

These applications focus on the competitive market dynamics and drug performance, both from tactical and strategic standpoints. They are either designed as comparative studies between the subject drug and its competitors, or they focus solely on the activities of the subject drug in order to enhance its performance.

Brand-Level Patient Share: Before patient data, typical brand share applications focused on market share analysis based on dollar sales or prescriptions by using legacy datasets. However, because the value of a patient varies between therapies, the calculation of the number of patients from sales and prescription data cannot be determined accurately. A top-to-bottom approach starting with total sales or scripts in order to derive the number of patients makes a lot of assumptions and has a lot of caveats.

Sales data does not offer an accurate reflection of the true share of patients by product due to the pricing differences of the drugs in a market, especially in terms of the higher-priced newer drugs when compared to older drugs in the same class and generic drugs. The value of a patient to manufacturers varies accordingly. Expensive therapies can easily outperform low-cost therapies even with a small share of patients. Prescription data comes closer to providing a true patient share, but the new prescription measures cannot differentiate between a new patient and a patient with a new script from the doctor continuing on therapy. As a result, it took the introduction of patient data and the patient ID to resolve the latter issue and allow analysts to determine patient share.

Patient share also provides better insights to market growth and trends. Dollar growth due to price increases is easily measurable, but growth due to shifting patients from low to high-cost therapies affects the dollar amount of the market size measured without any change in the number of patients. Market unit growth analysis is more insightful, but the incompatibility of units for different drugs makes it difficult to calculate the true change. Brand share analysis based on the number of patients is important because it allows the bottom-up building of models, an invaluable process used in forecasting. By using dosing data, one may calculate the unit and dollar measures.

The share of patients may vary by the type of patient who is influenced by incentives and disincentives. For example, low-cost drugs may have a higher patient share in the cash-paying patient group, and Medicare patients may be more cost-sensitive than the third-party managed care patient population. Consequently, a study should consider its target patient population before selecting the most appropriate database.

Source of Business:
These applications allow analysts to track the precise number of patients who, on a monthly basis, initiate, continue with their existing therapy, switch, add, restart, or discontinue a therapy. More specifically, the analysis provides counts of prescriptions and patients for a given drug therapy, in reference to a previous time period, and breaks the counts down based on the various patient behaviors. As such, these analyses provide a window into understanding the source of a brand's business, and can further be used to understand the effectiveness of various marketing and sales activities, as well as the overall performance of the brand.

For chronic diseases, a patient initiates therapy for the first time at some point in their life and follows the course of treatment through until such a time that they discontinue therapy entirely. The patient usually starts with a particular drug and continues with it until the drug is perhaps substituted with another or, if the circumstances require it, a second drug is added to their therapy. Patients may temporarily stop their therapy and re-initiate it at a later time with the same drug, or a new drug altogether.

The source of business analysis between therapies is important to the manufacturers because it has a direct impact on the demand for their products. For a product to grow at a healthy pace, not only it must be able to maintain its existing base of patients, but it must also claim a proportional share of the new patients entering the market. It is inevitable that a product will lose a number of patients to competing products, but at the same time it must claim a number of patients from other products to substitute for those losses. For growing markets, the patients starting therapy will outnumber the patients discontinuing therapy; in this, one may observe an increase in the overall number of prescriptions and patients. Below is a list of relevant concepts to the analysis.

- **Continuing:** Patients continuing therapy on the study drug
- **New Therapy Starts:** Patients new to the therapy this period with no prescriptions for the same drug in the look-back period
- **Add on:** Patients continuing their current therapy but adding a new drug to their therapy for the treatment of the same disease
- **Re-initiated:** Patients starting therapy again on the same study drug after discontinuing for a length of time longer than the refill grace period
- **Switched to:** Patients discontinuing an alternative therapy and starting therapy on the study drug
- **Switched from:** Patients starting therapy on an alternative drug having discontinued therapy on the study drug

A brand's new business is the sum of new therapy starts, therapy add-ons, and switched-to patients. Figure 18 demonstrates the composition of new business for five brands. Continuing patients and patients reinitiating therapy represent the brands existing business. The difference between the switched-to and switched-from is the net gain or loss of the brand's switching activity. Re-initiation analysis of patients that temporarily discontinue their therapies looks into whether the patient restarts therapy on the same drug or is switched to an alternative therapy.

TIP: *The definitions of the above terms may vary between vendors and manufacturers and must therefore be reviewed as part of the study's business rules before the initiation of a study.*

Source of business studies usually analyze a dynamic sample or cohort of patients for the most recent reporting month for the aforementioned changes with their drug utilization. The study requires a look-back period for determining if the patient was treated in the past to qualify them as new or re-initiated patients. This is done by looking for any previous prescriptions associated with the disease. Patients are said to have discontinued their therapy if they fail to refill their prescription for a specified period of time or grace period. Refills within the grace period will qualify the patient as a continuing patient. Both the look-back and grace periods are determined by various business rules.

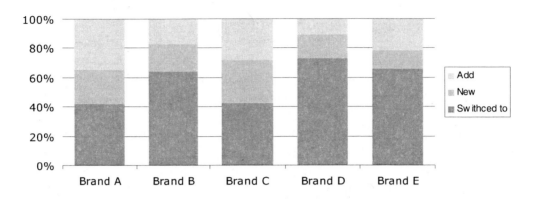

Figure 18: *Sources of new business by brand – Courtesy of IMS Health*

Patient data addresses the shortcoming of the legacy prescription products in that legacy prescription products are unable to capture truly new scripts. The NRx measure was inflated every time a patient refilled a prescription at a different pharmacy than the original fill or refilled with a new prescription slip from the physician. Consequently, the calculation of refills was understated by the number of erroneous new scripts. Patient data captures the treatment patterns of each unique patient distinctly, and therefore eliminates miscounting.

A source of business analysis for purely retail drugs requires a database with a healthy sample of pharmacy claims. For markets with a mix of retail and physician's office or hospital-administered drugs, a closed-panel or an integrated database of pharmacy, professional, and hospital claims is required. In the event that non-drug therapies exist in the market, a more comprehensive study would include these therapies in the analysis.

Although the analysis counts the patient movements between therapies precisely, it does not explain the reasons for the movements. In fact, because drug samples are not captured in the data, it is not possible to tell what drug a patient was definitively started on. This is usually because the patient was started on another drug with samples before the patient was put on their first prescription therapy. Physicians and patients are typically reluctant to make changes to a therapy to which the patient responds well. Switching often is the result of step-up or step-down therapies due to worsening or improvement of the patient's condition. Switching may also take place because of adverse effects, allergy reactions, a new therapy that has demonstrated a better efficacy or a better toxicity profile, reimbursement, etc. Physicians discontinue a patient's therapy when the patient is cured or when the symptoms have reached trivial levels. Patients, on the other hand, may prematurely discontinue their therapies against the advice of the doctors often because of economic reasons, a lack of perceived efficacy, or due to a misunderstanding of their own disease or the role of treatment.

This is critical information for the manufacturer. Yet, this is another example of claims data stating facts without being able to explain them. These questions currently require the use of primary market research to answer. EMR data has the potential of changing this in the future. Drug sample data could provide a better insight into therapy initiation and switching. Physician notes and the documentation of adverse affects and allergies could provide answers for the switching patterns post-initiation.

Physician Segmentation and Targeting: Segmentation is used extensively by pharmaceutical manufacturers to group their targets (for marketing purposes) based on certain characteristics ultimately associated with value and potential. Segmentation, traditionally, was done using legacy sales and script data, and was occasionally supplemented with some attributes from external databases in an attempt to identify account behavior patterns. The target of the activity was typically either the account or the prescriber.

The most common metric used was the prescriber's total script volume (TRx) for a particular product, or for all of the products in the same class; the metric was used as a measure of the physician's overall influence. Even though it was understood that the new script (NRx) measure did not equate to a measure of new patients, it was used as a proxy in the segmentation to represent the physician's ability to generate new business. For new product launches, where early adoption of the product by physicians is critical, analysts looked to classify physicians based on their propensity to adopt use of a new drug early, and thus, created the labels of early adopters, laggards, etc. That was done by using the same class (or even unrelated classes) of products and looking for the time lapsed between the launch of the product and the time of a physician's first filled script for the new product.

The payer's influence was a commonly used metric in the segmentation. The physician's case load by type of coverage, managed care, Medicaid or cash paying patients, or type of plan (HMO, PPO, IPA, etc.), were measurable metrics in script data. Other attributes used in the segmentation outside the script data included age and sex of the physician and other personal traits and characteristics, such as friendliness, their perception of technology, etc. These attributes were usually collected by using surveys.

With patient data, these concepts are still valid to a great degree, but patient data presented new opportunities to improve upon the segmentation applications through the use of new attributes that were previously not found in the script data. The presence of the patient ID in the data allows for the distinction of unique patients. Script data, sourced from the same claims data, is an aggregated dataset at the physician level that eliminates the patient ID attribute.

The ability to identify (true) new patients now eliminates the need to use the imprecise NRx metric in segmentation, and measures more precisely the physician's ability to drive new business. When put in perspective with the physician's TRx activity, it helps identify high-volume physicians with relatively low new patient or new to brand prescriptions: a sign that marketing resources are being overspent on those doctors. Conversely, physicians who would typically not receive much attention because they do not write a large number of prescriptions (but start a number of patients on a relevant therapy) may now be viewed as higher-value targets. Figure 19 demonstrates the breakdown of the traditional NRx measure in prescription data (left chart) to its actual components in patient data (right chart).

By using the patient ID, analysts can capture product switching, a measure associated with the physician's propensity to try new therapies. With script data this could be measured vaguely by the number of drugs in the class prescribed by the physician and the by number of new scripts for each product. Switching allows analysts to precisely measure movements between drug therapies and the order in which they took place. The sequence the drugs are prescribed typically reveals the physician's drug preferences for first, second, or subsequent lines of therapy. Switching away from the subject drug is of particular interest to the manufacturer for the purpose of defending against the erosion of the patient base of its drug. Manufacturers now have the opportunity to identify and segment doctors who are switching patients away from their drugs and to develop the right targeting and messaging strategies.

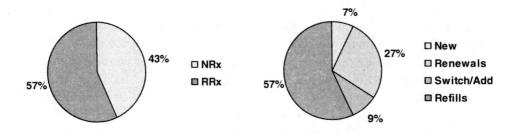

Figure 19: *Traditional Rx vs. patient data – Courtesy of Verispan LLC*

Another opportunity lies in segmenting physicians based on the severity of the patient case load. The severity of a patient can be determined by the amount of healthcare services they consume, measured in terms of encounters, procedures, testing, drug utilization, etc. Severe patients are usually on higher dosages of the drug; they may also be more compliant and persistent, which would set them apart as higher-value patients. With patient data, the managed care influence can be better weaved into the segmentation. Reversals, prior authorizations, and patient co-pays could all potentially be brought into the analysis to further enhance the results.

While script data enabled the segmentation of retail drugs by physician, it has absolutely no coverage of non-retail drugs. By bringing professional claims into physician segmentation, it is possible to introduce new variables like procedures to traditional segmentation. Medical claims allow one to resolve the indication issue for multi-indicated drugs before the segmentation so that physicians are targeted by the right sales force. Without medical claims, analysts must use the physician's specialty, product form, and strength as proxies for indication.

Pharmacy claims, like prescription data, provide significant physician coverage for targeting purposes. With professional claims, however, analysts can now link a physician directly to office drug utilization. Previously, the only way to establish that link was indirectly through DDD and Source Non-Retail drug sales data, and physician-to-account affiliations, without conclusive evidence in any case of the physician being responsible for the administration of the drug. Although professional claims databases do not capture the whole physician universe, the identification of even some of the physicians represents a significant improvement for targeting.

Hospital targeting has traditionally been based on the drug's sales volume to the hospital, taken together with physician-to-hospital affiliations and the physician's specialty, to narrow down the potential targets, though it has been without any further indication of a physician's influence. Procedure counts from hospital discharge databases are often used as a way to split sales by indication for drugs with multiple indications, or as a measure of potential where drug sales are inefficient. Hospital claims capture the attending and operating physician and up to two other physicians, whose role may not be clarified. In reality, the physicians on the claim may not be exclusively assigned to the care of the patient, and other physicians may be potentially involved in the care of the patient. Physician data from hospital claims may be used for targeting, assuming one understands certain caveats and the limitations of the assumptions made about their influence.

Physician segmentation and targeting are applications that require full visibility of the treatment universe of the physicians for the best results. Therefore, suitable patient databases for these applications are very large sample databases which capture as many physicians as possible. Physicians not visible in the data may not be assigned segment and target values. Pharmacy claims data is more likely to capture the entire universe of physicians, mainly because the sample sizes are larger and because the physician is more likely to be captured through the multiple collection points. Professional claims data samples are pretty sizable now.

However, they have less of a chance of capturing the entire universe of physicians because fewer physicians submit electronic claims. Consequently, when medical claims are used in the targeting, the results may be suboptimal.

Patient Segmentation: With claims data, an opportunity to segment the patient has arisen by looking at the patient characteristics. Based on their profiles, patients represent a certain opportunity for the manufacturers. This opportunity may be non-existent for patients whose profiles make them unsuitable for a particular treatment, but may exist for other patients who are between a minimum and a maximum value of disease severity, dosing and other factors. This exercise is important to manufacturers who are looking to extend their influence beyond the physician and closer to the patient.

The ultimate goal of patient segmentation is to cluster patients based on an assessment of their total healthcare service utilization; this includes both medical and drug use. Healthcare service utilization is typically a function of the severity of illness. Patients with more severe forms of the disease tend to utilize more healthcare services than less severe patients. Consequently, illness severity becomes a key consideration in the segmentation process.

Utilization can be measured both in terms of service encounters and treatments. Physician office visits, ER visits, hospitalization, nursing home stays are all examples of encounters. The procedures, rehabilitation services, lab tests, imaging, and prescription drugs all fall into the treatment category.

The first step in the segmentation process is to score the patient on the quantity of services, treatment utilization, and various markers of illness severity. Such scoring is necessary because the data elements in patient data are usually incompatible pieces of information that must somehow be normalized and given weight factors so that they can be aggregated to create an overall score. The scoring is based on individual patient data attributes that are captured in claims data or composite attributes. Assigning a number of points to a physician visit and tallying the number of points for all visits would be an example of an individual attribute score. Composite attributes are defined by the combination of two or more data elements. For example, the calculated total of the number of drug administrations times the unit dose is a composite attribute.

Once the scoring variables have been defined, a computerized statistical process performs the evaluation on a selected cohort of patients. The process eliminates any outliers and clusters the patients into a number of buckets. This is an iterative process until the results are optimized for the number of clusters and the number of patients in each cluster. As each cluster represents a segment, the idea is to have a manageable number of segments with each segment having neither too many nor too few patients.

Finally, once the clusters have been defined, clusters must be characterized by creating the descriptive statistics that would allow the data user to understand, at a granular level, the differences in the segments. Ultimately, these differences point to differential patient values, overall illness severity and most importantly, potential unmet treatment needs. Figure 20 demonstrates the results of a patient segmentation study. *Segment-A* consists of relatively older patients, has high level of comorbidities, and is more likely to see specialists. *Segment-B* has medium level of comorbidities but the highest level of healthcare encounters. *Segment-C* represents the youngest segment, has the lowest level of comorbidities, and infrequent healthcare encounters.

	Segment A	Segment B	Segment C
Mean Age (years)	53.9	51.7	46.0
Age Categories			
0-34	4.5%	8.5%	19.9%
35-54	48.1%	49.5%	49.4%
55-64	32.4%	28.3%	22.0%
65+ years	15.0%	13.7%	8.7%
Gender (%)			
Female	72.6%	71.7%	71.0%
Male	27.4%	28.3	29.0%
Physician Specialty (%)			
PCP	15.5%	18.1%	23.2%
Rheumatology	41.7%	40.3%	30.6%
Surgery	3.9%	3.5%	3.7%
Others/Unknown	38.9%	38.1%	42.5%
Charlson Index (0-16)	1.6	1.4	1.3
Comorbidities (%)	50.5%	42.5%	36.4%
Medical Procedures (%)	88.3%	87.0%	85.7%
All Hospital Stays (Mean)	0.2	0.4	0.1
ER Visits (Mean)	0.4	1.0	0.3
Office Visits (Mean)	11.2	23.9	6.2
	Below Avg	Average	Above Avg

Figure 20: *Patient segmentation – Source: IMS Health*

DTC/DTP Programs:
Direct-to-consumer (DTC) programs are marketing programs that manufacturers have used for the promotion of their products. These programs use television, radio, newspaper and popular magazine ads, and

more recently, the internet to reach the patient directly. Traditionally, by using general patient profiling information, manufacturers developed their messages and selected the most applicable media and markets to air the ads. Manufacturers relied on general sales and prescription trends to evaluate the effects of the programs. The area where the advertisement aired was expected to show increased sales and script activity.

Conceptually, the process followed the right steps, though the whole process lacked precision when it was first implemented. The patient profiles were based on primary market research with a limited sample and little factual data, and so was the messaging that was based on those profiles. The program evaluation that was based on sales and script data could not distinguish between patients who had received the message versus patients in the same market that had not. Message testing had to take place at a geographic market level, with local markets contrasted against other geographical markets (or the rest of the nation) because that was the lowest level of analysis that prescription and sales data could deliver.

Patient data did not replace any of that; instead, it helped improve the process in terms of patient profiling, message development, targeting the right audience, and capturing and evaluating results by introducing an unprecedented level of precision. Manufacturers can now test their message with a control group of patients and observe therapy initiations and drug switching in comparison to the general patient population.

The most notable difference, however, was the introduction of direct-to-patient (DTP) programs. Another form of DTC programs, DTP is not aimed at the general target patient population, as would a television ad attempt, but instead directs its message towards specific patients. Messages and promotional material are delivered directly to the large number of patients responding to the manufacturer's web site, mail or phone campaigns. Patients in search of disease or drug information usually volunteer their identity and details of their medical condition in exchange for the information. This was something they could do previously on a smaller scale by completing the return mail information cards in magazines, returning coupons, or by calling the toll-free numbers offered by radio and television ads. The phone and mail cards are still in use today for patients without access to the internet. However, the efficiency of the internet gave a tremendous boost to the patient-manufacturer communication.

Manufacturers are now able to combine the clinical and consumer profiles of these patients from claims and consumer databases for the purposes of patient segmentation. The key benefit of the consumer and clinical profile combination is a much improved patient segmentation based on location, age, sex, disease severity, healthcare utilization, treatment profiles, adherence status, and benefit considerations, coupled with income level, spending habits, affluence, lifestyle, education, etc. This type of segmentation allows marketers to develop more precise messages and targeting, and to subsequently test them using test and control groups that are defined from the same pool of patients.

Consumer profiles are generally not subject to any personal information protection regulations and are easily compiled and searched by using a consumer's social security, name, address, and age. Consumer databases are widely available in the market. However, the patient's clinical data is protected by HIPAA guidelines, and as a result, the matching of the identified patient from the manufacturer's database to the vendor's de-identified patient data has to happen anonymously. This is done by first encrypting the identity of the patients in the manufacturer database through the data vendor's encryption algorithm, and then by matching the patients through the use of the encrypted attributes. The encryption of the identified patients is performed by a third-party vendor so that no single entity holds copies of both the encrypted and unencrypted identities, which would immediately be a violation of the HIPAA patient confidentiality rules.

Evaluating the effect of a program can be done by directly tracking the claims data of the subject patients for treatment changes, which measures patient acquisition or conversion to the brand in addition to improved adherence, etc. In addition, based on the segmentation scheme, an algorithm evaluates and places newly signed-up patients into the defined segments based on predefined characteristics. Patients can then receive the appropriate messages though custom promotional material.

Epidemiology

Epidemiology is principally dedicated to monitoring the occurrence and causes of disease. Its main goal is to track the new disease population (incidence) and total disease population (prevalence), and to further study the severity of disease, the patient characteristics, the burden of the disease, services consumed, and uses of medication for the treatment of the disease. Epidemiology uses data as a strategic tool for planning and evaluating measures for disease prevention and management of the existing patient population. Epidemiological data has traditionally been widely available, mainly due to early government agency initiatives to track health risks in the general population. These initiatives were matched with private and non-profit organization initiatives that further increased the surveillance of diseases.

The sources of epidemiological data vary, though they often include surveys, national registries, death records, hospital discharge data, etc. For commercial purposes and for use in the pharmaceutical and medical industries in general, data vendors tapped into these sources to compile tabular databases that could be queried for a disease in order to get patient counts, including counts by disease stage. Patient data, claims in particular, presented the pharmaceutical manufacturer with the opportunity to use evidence-based data in studying the epidemiology of diseases. Epidemiological data is important for the manufacturer from the market size, patient characteristic, disease severity, and consumption pattern standpoints. Commercial applications of the data include uses in sales forecasting and market opportunity assessment. Clinical applications of the data include the study of diseases, planning new research, and product development.

Patient Population: This is the key metric of any epidemiology database. The fundamental question is how many new and existing patients of a particular disease there are amongst the target population. Patient data allows researchers to estimate that number from large samples of claims data. The estimates may be based on patient diagnosis or treatment.

NOTE: It should be noted here that epidemiological data based on claims relies solely on the physician's differential diagnosis, which may not necessarily be pathologically confirmed. The data quality standards in studies using claims data may therefore be lower than systematic epidemiological studies. Conversely, due to the exponentially larger sample size, they may actually have less patient population bias than many epidemiological studies using more rigorous data collection, particularly for smaller diseases.

For diagnosis-based estimates, the key data attribute that qualifies the patient in the count is the diagnosis code found in the medical claims databases. The diagnosis is based on the very granular ICD-9 codes, and describes the disease precisely, which then allows for the grouping and sub-grouping of patients. Treatment-based estimates using claims data focus only on the treated population with drug therapies. Patients are qualified by the presence of prescription claims or medication possession for predefined medications. The medication possession accounts for patients without a script during a specific time period of observation, but who also have some quantity of the drug left from a previous time period. Treatment-based estimates provide counts of patients with a specified disease who are on certain types of medications. The caveat with these estimates is that a drug treatment that is not qualified by a diagnosis is subject to error due to off-label use and multiple drug indications. The longitudinal nature of claims data allows researchers to estimate incidence of a disease over a specified period of time by validating that the patient, historically, was neither diagnosed nor treated.

Ultimately, the manufacturer is interested in projections to the target population from the claims database sample. Projections are possible when the composition of the database is known, or in simple terms, when what the database represents is clear. Given the nature of the various claims data products discussed earlier, existing claims databases may be projectable to one of the following population groups: national, insured, third party managed care, Medicare, or self-insured employer.

Open panel databases usually capture all types of patients and can be projected to the total population. Commercial applications normally target the entire US population and make use of these databases. Closed-panel databases capture specific patient types, and consequently their projectability is often limited to those populations.

Diagnosed vs. Treated:

This application estimates the number of patients treated for a disease in relation to the number of patients diagnosed with that disease. The untreated population, or the difference between the diagnosed and treated patients, is of interest to the manufacturer from a business opportunity standpoint. By definition, when using claims data, a treated patient meets certain diagnosis criteria and was prescribed a therapy with evidence that the therapy was followed. An untreated patient meets the diagnosis criteria in the data and may or may not have been prescribed a therapy, but there is no evidence in the data for any therapy. Therefore, the first condition that must be met in these studies is the existence of relevant diagnosis codes.

Treatment options for different diseases vary. The most common treatment method is medicating. The therapy spectrum also includes surgery, radiation, rehabilitation, phototherapy, and psychotherapy. The definition of "treated" includes literally all possible therapies. Therefore, a study should take into consideration all treatment modes. Treatment distinctions between drug and non-drug therapies (and further, between classes and product brands) lead to the full mode of therapy analysis discussed previously.

Closed-panel databases are best positioned for these applications because they capture all of the patient's medical and pharmacy claims. The time lag of these databases should not be a consideration in most cases, except for markets with recent significant developments where the delayed data will not reflect the effects of these events. One caveat with these databases is that the price-sensitive, uninsured patients are not represented in the data. Price sensitivity leads not only towards lower-cost therapies, but also to higher rates of untreated patients. The Medicare population, once considered a price-sensitive group, is more likely now to be treated, although the path of treatment patterns may be different than those observed in other covered groups. Open-panel databases cannot guarantee the capture of all of the patient's claims for any period of time, and has a good chance of misclassifying patients.

Claims data does not account for drug samples and OTC drug therapies; consequently, they understate the percent of treated patients. OTC treatments are not usually given much importance, which ignores the fact that many OTC products were previously prescription drugs that have demonstrated exceptionally safe profiles. EMR data has the potential of changing the definition of "treated" in the future with the capture of OTC drugs, alternative therapy, drug sampling, and prescribed-but-not-followed treatment data.

Disease Staging: This is one of the more complex patient data applications because the data is not fully supportive, yet it is of high value to specialties such as oncology. Disease staging clusters clinically homogeneous patients who require similar treatment and have similar expected outcomes. Disease stages are closely associated with specific drug therapies, regimens, and lines of therapy. Therefore, they have a direct impact on the manufacturer's revenue. Below are the standard definitions of disease staging:

Stage 0:	The patient is predisposed to a risk of the disease but has no symptoms yet
Stage 1:	A disease without complications
Stage 2:	The disease has local complications
Stage 3:	The disease has systemic complications or disease occurs in multiple sites
Stage 4:	The disease involves the risk of death

Disease staging is defined by its topology, etiology, and pathophysiology, or in layman's terms, where it takes place, why it occurred and what abnormalities and physiological disturbances it has caused, respectively. Staging is a function of disease severity, which in its ultimate state is the risk of causing organ failure or death. The more severe the level of disease is, the more advanced its stage will be. Generally, patient treatment for lower stages is initiated with more cost-effective and safer drug therapies before progressing to costlier or riskier therapies.

Disease staging is applicable to all diseases and requires proper diagnosis and thorough testing to determine accurately. For most non-life threatening diseases, however, physicians will diagnose the disease without making a conscious effort to identify and record its stage. Cancer, being very life-threatening, is something of an exception because it requires very precise staging so that the appropriate treatment can be administered.

Claims data does not account for disease staging, and there is no attribute in these databases for that purpose. For most diseases, therapy progression analysis by using claims data identifies (indirectly) the lines of therapy that can be associated with a disease stage. Early oncology staging applications, before EMR data, tried to exploit drug usage patterns in claims data in order to determine the disease stage. Armed with the knowledge of what drug regimens are used in different stages, analysts looked for a specific cancer diagnosis and tracked the number of patients on each regimen.

Staging, drug utilization, and dosing was what early EMR data was all about. The data comes from specialized EMR modules of oncology clinics. EMR systems do account explicitly for disease staging through the use of an actual stage field. However, the field is not consistently populated for patients and it is only found in a percentage of records. EMR systems also utilize data fields to capture the tumor, nodes, and metastasis status of the disease. Referred to as the TNM fields, when the values of the fields are examined in combination, a specific combination implies a specific disease stage.

One advantage of the use of the TNM fields over the stage field is that it avoids a weakness of staging: namely, that patients are staged once initially and continually referred to by that stage, even as their disease progresses. For example, a patient that was initially diagnosed with stage II cancer that later became metastatic should be referred to as a stage II patient with metastatic disease. TNM values, on the other hand, change over time with disease progression and can help identify longitudinally the patient's progressed disease stage.

Comorbidity Analysis:
Comorbidity is the presence of one or more diseases that exists at the same time with a primary condition. Comorbidities are important because they make the clinical management of patients more complex, as they influence their treatment and outcomes. Comorbidities deteriorate the prognosis of patients. Patients whose prognosis is too poor may not be able to tolerate therapy or may be denied a particular treatment. In addition, a would-be preferred therapy sometimes may be contraindicated due to comorbidities. Comorbidities often tend to increase with age and have an effect on patient survival.

Pharmaceutical manufacturers study comorbidities with the disease of interest in order to identify their impact on the use of their drugs. Specifically, there is a large focus on any advantages or disadvantages when compared to the competition, especially in relation to the performance of the drug in the presence of comorbidities. Next, the advantages and disadvantages are weighed to calculate opportunity or loss. The goal of the study is to determine the comorbidities of the highest risk and the patient populations associated with them. The studies usually measure the prevalence of comorbidities by age and sex.

Comorbidity analysis uses medical claims data to identify the primary and comorbid diagnoses and how frequently they occur. Typical reports provide frequency distributions of number of patients by number of comorbidities and type of comorbidity. Using pharmacy claims for these groups of patients, the drug utilization patterns can be compared to patients without comorbid conditions to estimate the impact of comorbidities on the drug of interest. A less precise method uses strictly pharmacy data to identify concomitant use of drugs. The drug classes used serve as a proxy for the diagnoses. The following chart demonstrates the comorbid conditions observed in the patient population with metabolic syndrome.

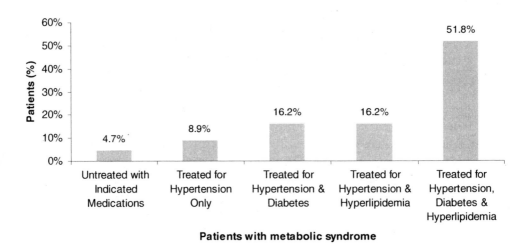

Figure 21: *Treatment utilization patterns – Source: IMS Health*

Closed-panel databases are well-positioned for these applications because of their ability to capture all of the diagnoses of a patient. EMR data, with its additional clinical data, has the potential of explaining comorbidities and concomitances better in the future.

Pharmacoeconomics & Outcomes

Pharmacoeconomics is part of the larger field of health economics that studies the costs, benefits and management of health care services. Pharmacoeconomics focuses on demonstrating the value of the manufacturer's drug to patients, payers, providers, and other stakeholders. This is done by measuring the economic impact of drugs in relation to the health outcomes and their benefits. Therefore, on one side of the equation, there are the economic outcomes, measured in terms of consumption of healthcare resources (direct costs), productivity costs (indirect costs), as well as quality of life, functional status and patient satisfaction (intangible costs), and on the other side, the clinical outcomes are measured in terms of changes in the health status of the patient.

Pharmacoeconomics plays a key role in the manufacturer's product pricing strategy and makes a good case for gaining formulary acceptance and reimbursement. It also plays a key role in the manufacturer's decision making with regard to product development and acquisition. Pharmacoeconomic studies are among the most powerful marketing instruments, as they help manufacturers differentiate their product from other branded and generic competing products.

Pharmacoeconomics combine cost, treatment and utilization, epidemiological, adherence, patient characteristic, and employer productivity data together with patient satisfaction, quality of life, patient preference, and functional effect of therapy data in order to demonstrate the cost and benefit relationships of therapies.

Burden of Illness: The burden of illness application is the cornerstone of pharmacoeconomics. It measures the cost of healthcare services to treat a particular disease from reimbursed claims. The costs are inclusive of all physician office visits, hospitalizations, rehabilitation, ER visits, procedures, and drugs used for the treatment. The analysis is usually based on the reimbursed amounts, and therefore, it reflects the cost to the payer and the patient.

Disease treatment involves a number of options. Drug therapies must demonstrate a reduced utilization of other healthcare services (such as procedures and hospitalization) against non-drug therapies. Within drug therapies for similarly priced therapies with potentially similar efficacy and similar indirect costs, patient satisfaction and small clinical profile differences are important differentiating factors. More expensive therapies are already assumed to have better efficacy, and must demonstrate better indirect and intangible cost profiles in addition to better outcomes.

The analysis is applicable to both acute and chronic diseases. For chronic diseases, the impact is typically measured in terms of average annual expenditures calculated from a cohort of patients. The studies calculate both total costs and cost by various categories, such as encounter costs, procedure costs, pharmacy costs, etc. Utilization and costs of the drug of interest are compared to its class and other classes of drugs used for the treatment of a disease, or to specific competing drugs. Patient characteristics are important to the analysis, as utilization varies by age and sex, comorbidities, etc. The type of coverage and plan design factor into the analysis as well, because they impact utilization patterns, and consequently, costs. Differences should be expected both within payers and plan types, i.e. PPO, HMO, etc. Geographic differences due to local cost factors are also considered in the analysis.

Claims data captures the direct costs of treatment and part of the clinical outcomes in terms of service utilization. Professional claims capture days off-work, subject to data input, which can be used to partially measure the indirect costs associated with productivity. However, this is not necessarily a complete count of lost work days, and the data may not be captured with any regularity. Furthermore, productivity has a subjective, unquantifiable component that isn't accurately measured by the number of work days. The costs for a given drug must be qualified by an indication which uses a diagnosis code. As dosing for different indications varies, so do the costs.

Closed-panel databases are most often used for burden of illness applications due to their tight integration of the patient's total care records. For accuracy, pharmacoeconomic applications require that every episode of care is accounted for. Open-panel databases, even though they are generally a better representation of the total patient population, cannot guarantee the inclusion of all of the patient's claims due to the way they are sourced. It is important to note that the type of cost figures captured in the database can affect the analysis. Databases may be reporting submitted charges, allowed charges, paid amounts, or all of the above. The preferable metric is usually the paid amount, unless otherwise specified in the study.

Outcomes:

Outcomes are the end results of health care services and interventions. The definition of outcomes is rather broad, and it includes both clinical and economic components. Clinical outcomes measure the physiological attributes of the patient, disease symptoms, clinical events, functional health, mortality, and the patient's overall experience. The economic outcomes are based on burden of illness analysis.

Outcomes studies are complex, with the majority of the data coming from several sources. Physiological measures, such as test results, are captured in patient lab data. Other measures, such as heart rate, blood pressure, and additional symptoms, are in the domain of EMR data. Clinical events like heart attack and stroke are captured in claims data from diagnosis and procedure attributes. Some mortality information can be captured through hospital discharge data.

However, not all outcomes are measurable with patient data. Functional health and patient experience data can be captured either by the physician or by using survey instruments. One such survey is the SF-36 Health Survey, a general short-form, multi-purpose survey. The survey measures both physical and mental attributes in eight key areas: physical functioning, role-physical, bodily pain, general health, vitality, social functioning, role-emotional and mental health. Another example of this type of survey is the Medicare Health Outcomes Survey. Disease-specific surveys are more effective, however, because the measure changes as a result of treatment. The challenge with survey data is in matching general population surveys to specific de-identified patient data. These surveys are better conducted by an entity with access to the unencrypted patient data, like the payer or the employer with a controlled group of patients.

Outcomes studies using claims data seek to understand the patterns of care and their impact on the patient's clinical profile. The studies contrast healthcare utilization for patients on a specific drug against patients on another drug or a class of drugs. The studies measure the cost of the therapy and the presence, absence, or frequency of medical encounters, ER and hospital visits, procedures, etc.

Closed-panel databases are most often used for outcomes studies for the same reasons discussed in the burden of illness. Given the data's limitations today, these studies have rather a limited focus. A comprehensive study would need to utilize lab results, surveys, claims, and EMR data. This is another area of opportunity for EMR data if it is ever successfully implemented.

Time Value of Patient: This application measures the manufacturer's economic benefit over time from the patient's use of the drug. This measure is relevant to the manufacturer's revenue projections. The value of the patient to the manufacturer is a function of the patient's average daily consumption of the drug. Usually estimated as an annual average, it is the product of the average annual product consumption times the price of the drug. The price of the drug used could be obtained from the product's wholesaler acquisition cost (WAC), or the manufacturer may apply a price calculated from gross or net sales.

Accounting for differences in dosing, patient value varies within segments of patients. The analysis, therefore, may use patient characteristics to identify value differences in patients based on age, sex, and disease severity. Dosing can also vary drastically between drug indications, and therefore, the calculated patient values should be specific to indications. The indication should be qualified with the presence of a diagnosis code. The time value of a patient is directly correlated to the patient's treatment adherence. Less compliant patients fill fewer scripts in a year and less persistent patients end their therapies early, both contributing to diminished values.

Patient value applications are applicable to both retail and non-retail drugs, and they use both pharmacy and professional claims data. Both open and closed-panel databases support these applications. Assuring continuous enrollment of the patient during the study period is important to the application. Closed-panel databases have a small advantage in that they account for all of the qualifying patients' records and the inclusion of enrollment data. Open-panel databases must determine patient enrollment by using look-back and look-forward periods. Open-panel databases must be used for the calculation of patient value in the price-sensitive segments of cash-paying and Medicare patients.

Health and Productivity: General health and productivity studies have focused on quantifying the overall impact of lost productivity due to health issues. Loss of productivity is attributed to loss of work due to disability, sick days, or simply by working at a reduced capacity and being less productive as a result. The

latter, also referred to as presenteeism, is often the result of the employee not being able to afford days off of work due to a lack of benefits. The loss of productivity is not always attributed to an employee's own health problems, but may also be attributed to employee's care for a family member as well.

Health and productivity applications that use patient data are more focused on the effects of various therapies on worker productivity, given that the health status of an employee is closely related to the loss of productivity. The basic premise here is that effective treatments improve worker productivity. A patient's productivity at work improves as their physical and mental functional state and satisfaction with their treatment improves. Productivity represents the indirect cost component of pharmacoeconomics, and manufacturers like to measure and associate these economic outcomes with the benefits of drug therapies to further demonstrate the value of their products.

These productivity studies are comparative studies that benchmark the period of time prior to treatment or another therapy. Key differentiators in these studies are the age of sub-populations, income, marriage status, and children. With a significant number of self-insured employers and millions of lives insured, the results of productivity studies are very important to employers looking for effective therapies in their plan benefit designs, prevention programs, disease management, etc., but also to manufacturers seeking formulary inclusion for their drugs.

The analysis considers the patient's drug utilization from the claims data and supplements that with employee absenteeism, disability days, workers compensation days, and employee demographics with income and marital status data sourced from employers. Health and productivity studies require complete medical and pharmacy patient data; although this is possible in all closed-panel databases, employer-sourced claims databases take advantage of the existing data reporting relationship with employers by simply supplementing the claims data with the additional employee data attributes.

Reimbursement Analysis:
Historically, reimbursement analysis has been based on the plan attributes found in prescription data. Because of inherent limitations, prescription data did not lend any more insight than a breakdown of the physician's script activity for a drug by plan, payer, or PBM. When plan formulary data from sources outside the script data was brought into the analysis, it explained how much of a brand's business with the prescriber was disadvantaged due to unfavorable formulary, and similarly, how a physician's prescribing habits were impacted by the plan formularies. The plan-covered lives, also from external sources, helped to quantify the extent of the plan's influence. Manufacturers could quantify the missed opportunity and take action with plans to change the status of their drugs with the plan's formulary.

Patient data did not affect this type of analysis much. However, a number of new data attributes and the capture of the patient's unique ID opened up new opportunities for the analysis of payer control and influence. The first opportunity came from the ability to closely observe the interaction of the pharmacy and the payer, and the analysis of rejected claims provided a new perspective on the payer's control. The second opportunity presented itself in the ability to capture more detailed information on the pharmacy-submitted and payer approved charges to quantify the patient's burden. Lastly, with the analysis of reversed transactions came the ability to measure the price sensitivity of patients based on their cost burden.

- **Claim Rejection Analysis** – This application analyzes the payer's reasons for rejecting the pharmacy claims submitted for adjudication. There are a few hundred pre-defined rejection reasons, however, the majority of them are due to edits and validations of the pharmacy input and system communication issues, with little relevance or impact to the manufacturer's business. The rejection reasons that interest the manufacturer are the ones that are related to the payer's control, such as benefit design, formulary, and prior authorizations.

Rejection Code	Rejection Reason	% of Rejections
79	Refill Too Soon	17.4%
76	Plan Limitation Exceeded	15.1%
70	Product/Service Not Covered	12.6%
69	Filled After Coverage Terminated	9.6%
88	DUR Reject Error	6.0%
75	Prior Authorization Required	5.2%
68	Filled After Coverage Expired	3.6%
65	Patient Is Not Covered	3.0%
73	Refills Are Not Covered	0.6%
41	Submit Bill To Other Processor Or Primary Payer	0.5%

Figure 22: *All market claims rejections by code – Source: Wolters Kluwer*

Rejection analysis is a payer or plan-level activity. High plan rejection activity signifies a business risk for the manufacturer, as rejected prescriptions are likely to be switched to prescriptions for competing products. The first step in the analysis is to determine which rejection codes are of interest and indicative of business issues. Ranked lists of payers or plans with high percentages of rejections identify the high-risk plans. Rejection reasons and counts are cross-tabulated to identify the most common reasons for rejection.

The rejections of the product of interest can be contrasted with competing products to determine if it is disadvantaged against its competitors. Figure 22 demonstrates the frequency of occurrence of important rejection reasons.

This analysis can be combined with formulary data from external databases to contrast the formulary position of a drug with a plan in order to better explain the payer actions. The manufacturer's course of action is usually a negotiation with the payers in an attempt to position the product more effectively in the plan formularies.

- **Claim Reversal and Price Sensitivity Analysis** – This application considers the reasons behind pharmacy-reversed transactions. After a prescription is adjudicated, the pharmacy proceeds to fill the prescription. If the patient does not claim or refuses the filled prescription, the pharmacy issues a reversal or cancellation to the payer to void the pending payment and re-stocks the drug.

   Most commonly, the prescription is refused by the patient due to cost considerations and high out-of-pocket expenses. The patient is then likely to accept a generic version of the drug at a lower cost, if one exists. Alternatively, the patient may accept a drug with a more favorable status in the insurance plan's formulary for a lower out-of-pocket cost, or choose not to fill the prescription at all. In any case of a reversal, the manufacturer of the original drug has incurred an opportunity loss that they would like to avoid in the future.

   Reversals occur more often with new prescriptions and the first fill. This is the moment when the patient decides if the out-of-pocket expense is acceptable to them. Patients may reconsider their out-of-pocket cost with every refill, but they are more likely to continue with the same therapy after the first fill. Patients are also likely to make changes at the beginning of a new coverage period if the benefit design has changed and if their cost share has increased.

   The patient's costs include an initial deductible they must meet, regardless of the product, before any payer contribution. Subsequently, a co-pay or co-insurance is applicable to any prescription. Co-pays come with tiers. A common three-tier co-pay would require a lower patient contribution for generic drugs, a medium payment for branded products, and a higher contribution for premium, high-cost therapies. Co-insurance requires the patient to contribute a pre-specified, fixed percentage of the overall prescription cost. Some plans come with benefit maximums where, once exceeded, the patient must assume the entire cost of the prescription.

   During the deductible phase, a lower-cost drug is more appealing to the patient. Because the patient is assuming the entire cost, the preferred choice is often to defer meeting the deductible. During the co-pay phase, drugs in the higher co-pay tiers will likely be disadvantaged, as are more expensive drugs with patient co-insurance. Higher-cost drugs will be definitely at risk in the benefit maximum phase.

Price sensitivity analysis measures the patient's propensity to choose a lower-cost therapy at different price points. The analysis focuses on reversed and subsequent transactions to compare the patient's out-of-pocket costs of each transaction. Figure 23 demonstrates that patients with high out-of-pocket costs on average switched to a much cheaper alternative. The data gathered helps manufacturers take countermeasures in order to retain the customer. Usually, the recourse is found in payer contracting and volume rebates, which move the product to a more favorable formulary position in order to lower the patient's costs. Alternatively, manufacturers offer direct patient incentives like co-pay assistance, coupons for free prescriptions, etc.

	Avg. OPC* Paid Rx	Avg. OPC Reversed Claim	Avg. OPC Reversal Substitution	Avg. OPC Difference
Aciphex	$35.42	$88.19	$26.53	$56.48
Nexium	$31.48	$85.21	$23.73	$61.06
Omeprazol	$9.99	$36.30	$27.93	$3.95
Prevacid	$28.99	$85.05	$26.60	$43.78
Protonix	$30.35	$75.26	$24.17	$51.69

* Out-of-Pocket Cost

Figure 23: *Co-pay sensitivity analysis – Source: Verispan LLC*

- **Co-pay Analysis** - The co-pay is a control instrument utilized by the payers to manage the costs associated with the reimbursement of drug therapies. One feature that makes pharmacy plans attractive to customers is drug choice. However, not all therapies cost the same, and to discourage excessive patient use of high-cost therapies, payers institute higher co-pays for more expensive therapies. Co-pays for the same drug in different payer plans will vary based on the plan premium. A higher premium plan would have lower co-pays, and consequently, co-pay becomes one of the elements of plan design.

  Payers seek to mitigate some of the risk of the high-cost therapies through manufacturer rebate programs. Rebate programs based on volume are maximized when a high concentration of business comes through a smaller number of drugs, which the formulary controls. Drugs under contract are then assigned to a lower co-pay tier while non-contracted drugs are assigned to higher co-pay tiers (or are not included in the formulary, and therefore, not rcimbursed).

Co-pay is of particular interest between other payer cost control measures. Deductibles, co-insurance and benefit maximums all favor drugs in lower-cost tiers. Higher-cost therapies are competitively priced against each other by manufacturers, and the above measures have little effect on drug choice within the same pricing tier. The co-pay is the only measure that can shift the powers between similarly priced drugs, and as a result, is a more important cost control measure.

Co-pay analysis looks not only into differences between lower and higher-cost therapies, but also between similarly priced therapies. Large co-pays disadvantage not only products within a class, but also entire classes against other classes. The analysis assesses the entire competitive landscape at the plan level, as co-pays tie specifically to plans.

The co-pay analysis is complicated by the fact that the co-pay is more frequently reported in the 'Patient Pay Amount' as part of the overall patient out-of-pocket expense, and less frequently in its dedicated 'Amount of Co-pay/Co-insurance' field. The reported amount in that case may include deductible costs, over the coverage-maximum amounts, and premiums due to product selection. Even though the co-pay or co-insurance for a product would be expected to be constant for a patient, the sum of all of the above in any combination results in out-of-pocket expenses varying widely.

The analysis is usually a distribution of ranges of co-pay amounts that determines what patients typically pay for the drug. Outlier amounts usually include more than the co-pay or co-insurance. The analysis may also provide the average co-pay of competing drugs within a plan to highlight a product's advantaged or disadvantaged position. In addition, the average co-pay of a brand across plans highlights the differences between plan positioning.

Medicare Part-D Coverage Gap Analysis: The introduction of Medicare drug coverage provided manufacturers with a new opportunity, because elders and other Medicare eligibles previously without coverage could now afford to fill prescriptions that they would otherwise have avoided filling. With that came the need for the manufacturer to understand how patients respond to the changes from one phase of the coverage to another, this being a very price-sensitive patient group. The Medicare population is an important market for the manufacturer because of the high incidence of chronic diseases in this segment.

Medicare drug coverage varies from the typical managed care plan, where the patient enters a deductible phase before moving into a co-pay or co-insurance phase and before they reach a potential over-the-benefit-maximum phase. With standard Medicare Part-D coverage, patients enter a deductible phase, then move into a 25% co-insurance phase and continue into a no-coverage phase, often referred to as the "donut hole," before they reach the catastrophic coverage limit with a low co-pay or co-insurance. The deductible, co-insurance, "donut hole," and catastrophic range limits are adjusted periodically by Medicare. The 2007 limits are a $265 deductible, $266-$2,400 for co-insurance, and $2,401-$5,451.25 for no coverage. Part-D coverage is not actually provided directly by Medicare, but through private insurers. Although the above represent minimum coverage standards set by Medicare, health plans may offer alternatives to the standard Part-D plans, some of which provide co-insurance or co-pays without the "donut hole" benefit phase, or they may provide low co-pay generic coverage through the donut hole.

Medicare offers three other plan options to patients depending on their poverty level: dual-eligible patients below the poverty level, patients within 101-135% of the federal poverty level (FPL), and patients within 135-150% of federal poverty level. These plans either have no deductible, or the deductible is very low. The plans lack the no-coverage phase and instead, patients have a very low co-pay or a moderate co-insurance for the entire range between the deductible and the catastrophic phase, depending on their poverty level. Dual-eligibles are patients who are entitled to Medicare Part A and/or Part B and are eligible for some form of Medicaid benefit. The poverty level (or more accurately, the poverty guidelines) is defined in terms of income by the department of health and human services, and is adjusted annually based on price changes through the most recent complete fiscal year.

Medicare Part-D analysis focuses mostly on the standard benefit patient population, which is not eligible for any subsidies. For the other three groups, the out-of-pocket cost of the drugs is rather low, especially for the dual-eligible and the 101-135% of FPL group. The analysis tracks patients and their consumption habits as they move through the various phases of their coverage. During the first three phases of the coverage, the patient's price sensitivity greatly affects their choice of drugs, as the patient's share of the cost is high, even in the co-insurance phase. Analysis focuses on the "donut hole" or the gap in coverage between the phases of initial benefit and catastrophic coverage. It is during the "donut hole" phase that patients may make decisions to discontinue certain medications and/or switch to less expensive alternatives. In the catastrophic phase, however, price sensitivity is no longer an issue. By then, the patient has settled into their therapy with less chance of switching. The analysis may involve a drug of interest, multiple competitors, or the market as a whole for each benefit group.

The main purpose of the analysis is to identify potential switching trends, as well as the compliance and persistence of patients entering the "donut hole" phase. The analysis measures potential shifts from branded to generic products, the products patients switched to, and the percentage of patients who discontinue their therapies. The analysis also looks more closely into how many patients restart their therapies in the catastrophic phase. Age demographic analysis may be used to capture the severity of patients by age group.

Another key activity of the process is to assess how many patients reach the "donut hole" and catastrophic phases over time. One way to do that is to run cumulative patient and payer totals of pharmacy expenditures for all therapeutic areas for a cohort of patients who have good coverage in the database. The patient counts can then be projected to the total known Medicare Part-D enrollment. Standard benefit patients are deemed to have reached the "donut hole" phase once the accumulated pharmacy costs are equal to the lower range limit of $2,400, based on the 2007 figures. Similarly, they have reached the catastrophic phase once the cumulative pharmacy cost exceeds $5,451.25. The beneficiary side costs are referred to as true out-of-pocket costs, or "TrOOP." Dual-eligibles and the 101-135% of FPL patients can be identified by precisely matching co-pay amounts in the transactions to the co-pay amounts set for the fiscal year in combination with the total pharmacy spend.

The analysis also measures the time it takes patients to move through the "donut hole" phase and into the catastrophic benefit phase. This depends on the severity of a patient's health, the cost of their therapies, and the number of medications they take. Patients with co-morbid conditions on multiple or higher-cost medications will move through the "donut hole" faster. Figure 24 demonstrates the percent of patients in each coverage phase several months out from the beginning of the coverage period. Other metrics measure the average monthly spend, average cumulative spend, and the number of medications of patients.

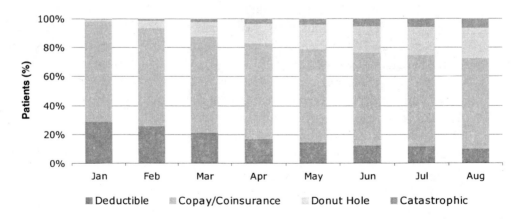

Figure 24: *Patients by coverage phase – Source: Wolters Kluwer*

The general impact of Medicare Part-D to the overall pharmaceutical expenditures can be assessed by using the projected legacy prescription and plan data. The data can be used to measure the magnitude of the Medicare business, the market growth due to the new Medicare business, and the changes to Medicaid due to the shift of patients to the Medicare Part-D benefit. Patient data can also be used to identify differences between a payer's Medicare and a commercial business in terms of market share, co-pay, rejections, and substitutions.

Medicare Part-D analysis requires a sizable pharmacy claims database with good third-party managed care coverage, as Medicare Part-D is offered through commercial plans. Open and closed-panel databases with broad payer coverage are suitable for this analysis. Employer database coverage is limited to retired employees with company sponsored Part-D coverage.

Epilogue

It is clear from this discussion that when it comes to patient data, the industry is still evolving. The industry still has a lot to learn not only with EMR data, which is obviously in its earlier stages, but also with claims data, which has existed for a while and has been explored quite a bit. While EMR data opens new opportunities for the future, one can hardly make the case that we are done with claims data. There are still unexplored areas within claims data that have the potential to give us many new insights. Therefore, this is not a case of only pushing ahead, but also of making the most out of what we have today.

Certainly, every data vendor has a ways to go, even though they appear eager to push the limits. Of course, such lofty goals are not entirely in their control because, as is the case with EMR data, they cannot change the pace of development. Their eagerness is driven primarily by the fact that this is the field that offers the highest degree of opportunity for vendors, in spite of an already crowded market. While they must keep pace with the industry's progress, this is a great opportunity for vendors to focus on improving their assets, and at the same time, to set their future strategy.

Improving the current products entails doing a few things: improving data sample sizes, adding new data types, increasing the number of data elements, improving integration, and improving contracting. A larger sample does not always mean better data, because projections from different sample sizes can generate statistically identical results, depending on the level of projection. Above a minimum sample size, projections are not improved. However, progressively larger samples are required with progressively lower level projection detail. Such samples are required for targeting and compensation applications. Pursuing these kinds of applications with sub-optimal databases will not be successful. Sample size is also an issue with low patient counts in certain therapeutic areas. Sample expansion will unnecessarily expand optimal samples of other therapeutic areas. However, it will secure minimum requirements for others.

Limitations within data are usually inherent to the source and method of collection. Databases need not be restricted to certain data sources, nor to a certain collection method. Databases should be designed flexibly to integrate new data types so that certain aspects of the data are improved. For example, in the ability to add data for a patient type not represented in the database, or to add data elements to claims data from EMR. Equally important, a lack of visibility to certain data elements translates to an inability to deal with certain types of applications. When lack of visibility to data elements is tied to data sourcing issues and the confidentiality of those sources, working out a solution is almost impossible. Otherwise, it might be due to an oversight. Data elements that look trivial today may prove significant later. All of the above limitations have one thing in common: they are the result of data contracting. Data contracting should be the key priority of a vendor's data strategy. Vendors should be looking for data sources that provide maximum flexibility and data breadth.

Data integration is ultimately what glues the parts together, regardless of whether they are composed of similar data from different sources, different data from the same source, or different data from different sources. In the end, patient data is a collection of data components that, when put together, create a product. Integration is about being able to identify the same patient in data from different sources. The more misses, or the higher the "leakage" rate is, the smaller the usable study sample becomes, and thus requires more data to improve the integrated set.

A data strategy must take into consideration two important aspects: human capital and data assets. Current data products have their strengths and weaknesses. That, combined with intense competition, leads vendors to seek their niche in the market. Vendor specialization is beneficial for the manufacturer because it usually translates to a higher quality analysis. Vendors would have to decide if that strategy fits them in the long term, considering what the competition may look like in the years ahead.

As always, and particularly with this complex area of patient data, the human capital becomes a strategic issue, first because this area requires better-than-average data expertise to meet the customer's needs, and second, because this area is in need of visionaries to drive it forward and innovate with new solutions, new data applications, and new analysis. As it is usually the case with new and developing markets, both are in short supply until the market reaches some level of maturity.

Glossary

Acute Care: Care provided for the treatment of an immediate and severe episode of illness, the subsequent treatment of injuries related to an accident or other trauma, or during recovery from surgery. Acute care is usually provided in a hospital by specialized personnel using complex and sophisticated technical equipment and materials. Unlike chronic care, acute care is often necessary for only a short time.

Adverse Drug Reaction (ADR): A particular type of adverse effect sometimes associated with the use of different medications.

Adverse Effect: A harmful or abnormal result from a therapy or other medical intervention.

Allowable Charge: See Approved Charge

Approved Charge: The amount determined by a payer to be reasonable payment for a provider for covered services under a health plan including co-pays, co insurance and deductibles.

Assignment: A process in which a doctor or supplier agrees to accept the payer-approved charge as payment in full.

Beneficiary. The person eligible to receive, or already receiving benefits from a drug or medical plan.

Benefit: A covered item such as a pharmaceutical, device, supply, service, or procedure by a private insurance plan or public health program.

C-Codes: Are used exclusively to report services, drugs, biologicals, and devices eligible for transitional pass-through payments for hospitals, and for items classified in new-technology ambulatory payment classifications (APCs) under the Outpatient PPS (Prospective Payment System). They may not be used to bill under other Medicare payment systems.

Centers for Medicare & Medicaid Services (CMS): Formerly the Health Care Financing Administration (HCFA). The federal government agency part of the Department of Health and Human Services which oversees the states' administrations of Medicaid, while directly administering Medicare.

Chronic Care: Care provided to individuals with long standing, persistent diseases or conditions.

Claim Adjudication: The determination of payment for a medical claim based on the member's insurance benefits.

Claims Clearinghouse: An entity that receives, translates, standardizes and forwards healthcare transactions between providers, payers and other health care partners.

Claim Payment Amount: The amount paid to the provider excluding co-pays, co-insurance and deductibles.

Claims Switch: A claims clearinghouse the routes electronic healthcare transactions.

Co-insurance: The percentage of the payer-approved amount that is the responsibility of the beneficiary. Co-pay and co-insurance are forms of cost sharing between payers and beneficiaries.

Co-pay: The flat dollar amount payment made by the patient to a provider for a medical service or a drug prescription. Co-pay and co-insurance are forms of cost sharing between payers and beneficiaries.

Co-morbidities: Diseases occurring at the same time.

Compliance-Drug: The adherence of the patient to the dosing instructions of the physician.

Concomitance, Diagnosis: Diagnoses that are reported by the patient together during the same visit.

Concomitance, Product: Drugs in combination therapies used together to treat the same diagnosis.

Covered Services: The health care services and supplies that may be reimbursed pursuant to a health plan.

Deductible: An out-of-pocket amount the insured person must meet before the benefits of a health plan begin.

Diagnosis Related Groups (DRGs): A classification system that categorizes illness by diagnosis and treatment and used to pay a hospital or other inpatient provider for their services. The provider is paid a fixed set amount for each DRG regardless of the provider's actual cost. The group definitions are based on medical diagnosis, treatments, procedures, patient age and sex, presence or absence of significant co-morbidities or complications, discharge status, and other relevant criteria. The federal government uses DRGs to reimburse hospitals for care to Medicare subscribers.

Direct-to-Consumer (DTC): Promotional activities targeting directly the patient and include print ads, commercials, internet content, etc.

Direct-to-Patient (DTP): Promotional activities targeting directly the patient as a result of a direct communication between the patient and the manufacturer.

Disease Management: A process based on therapeutic guidelines that targets to improve the patient's total condition in order to prevent acute episodes.

Dose Titration: The process of optimizing the effects of a drug by gradually adjusting the patient dosing.

Drug Utilization Review (DUR): Also known as Drug Utilization Evaluation (DUE). The systematic review of drug use patterns for the purpose of reducing the cost of utilization, typically performed by a DUR committee. The review examines the number of prescriptions per patient per month and the average cost per prescription. DURs are commonly performed by MCOs, hospitals, and other payers for physicians, physician groups, medical specialties, retail pharmacies, employee groups and patients. DUR sanction or reward practitioners depending on performance.

Electronic Medical Records (EMR): The digitally organized medical history and care of patients accomplished with the use of practice management software systems.

Eligible Person: The person entitled to receive covered services pursuant to a health plan.

Episode of Care: Healthcare services for a specific condition during a specific period of time.

Federal Poverty Level (FPL): Poverty guidelines defined by the department of health and human services for determining financial eligibility for certain federal programs. They are updated each year to reflect price changes through the most recent complete fiscal year.

Final Action Claim: A paid claim with all final adjustments made.

Formulary: List of approved drugs that will be reimbursed by the payer. Open formularies promote the use of generic and preferred drugs; Closed formularies reimburse only for approved drugs and require prior approval for use of other drugs.

Group Practice: A group of physicians that engage in the coordinated practice of their profession in one or more group practice facilities, and who share common overhead expenses, medical and other records, and substantial portions of the equipment and the professional, technical, and administrative staffs. Group practices are formed primarily because of the need to lower costs and improve the ability to contract.

Health Outcomes Research: The measurement of the end results of particular health care practices and interventions.

ICD-9-CM Diagnosis Codes: World Health Organization International Classification of Disease, 9th revision with clinical modification. Universal coding method used to document the incidence of disease, injury, mortality and illness.

ICD-9-CM Procedure Codes: Supplement codes for therapy modes, surgery, radiology, laboratory, and other diagnostic procedures.

Incidence: The number of new cases of disease, infection, or some other event over a period of time in reference to the population in which they occur.

J-code: HCPCS level II procedure codes that describe the administration of injectable medications in the physician office.

Managed Care: Healthcare systems and techniques used to control the use of healthcare services. Includes a review of medical necessity, incentives to use certain providers, and case management.

Managed Care Plan: A health plan that provides comprehensive care in a cost-effective manner. It has a defined system of selected providers that contract with the plan and enrollees have a financial incentive to use participating providers.

Medicaid: Government entitlement program for the poor who are blind, aged, disabled or members of families with dependent children (AFDC). The program is federally aided but state-operated and administered and provides medical benefits for certain indigent or low income persons in need of health and medical care. States set their own standards for qualification.

Medicare: A federal program providing health insurance for people at the age of 65 and older, and for disabled people of all ages. It is funded by the federal government and administered by the Centers for Medicare & Medicaid Services (CMS). Beneficiaries are responsible for deductibles and co-payments.

Medicare Dual Eligibles: Patients who are entitled to Medicare Part A and/or Part B and are eligible for some form of Medicaid benefit.

Medicare Part A: Covers hospitalization, nursing home care, hospice and the services of a home health agency. Medicare reimburses for hospital inpatient care based on DRGs and hospital outpatient care on a cost basis. Part A services are financed by the Medicare HI Trust Fund, which consists of Medicare tax payments.

Medicare Part B: Supplemental medical insurance which covers beneficiaries for physician services, medical supplies, and other outpatient treatment. Beneficiaries are responsible for monthly premiums, co-payments, deductibles, and balance billing. Part B services are financed by a combination of enrollee premiums and general tax revenues.

Medicare Supplement Insurance: A private insurance policy that supplements Medicare benefits by covering some costs not paid for by Medicare that include deductibles, co-payments and in many circumstances, services excluded by Medicare such as outpatient prescription drugs.

Medication Possession Ratio (MPR): The ratio of the actual drug quantity dispensed during a specified period to the quantity of drug needed for continuous use in the same time period.

Medigap: See Medicare Supplement Insurance

Method of Payment: Refers to the reimbursement breakdown of a drug by payment type.

Morbidity: The extend of disease, injury and disability in a defined population expressed in rates of incidence and prevalence.

Multi-Specialty Group: A group of physicians from different medical specialties who work in the same group practice.

National Drug Code (NDC): Drug coding system, sort of a serial number for a drug. The components of the NDC number identify the manufacturer, product and pack size.

Outcome: The result of medical or surgical intervention or non-intervention.

Outcome Measurement: System used to track clinical treatment and responses to that treatment, including measures of mortality, morbidity, and functional status.

Outcomes Management: Methods implemented by payers and providers for managing care in a way that would produce the best outcomes. Using a database of outcomes experience, providers know better which treatment modalities result in consistently better outcomes for patients. Outcomes management often results in the development of clinical protocols.

Outpatient Care: Also referred to as ambulatory care, it is care given to a patient who is not bedridden.

Over-the-Counter (OTC): Drugs that do not require a prescription.

Payer: An entity that assumes the risk of paying for medical treatments and includes a managed care organization, an indemnity insurance, Medicare, Medicaid, an uninsured patient, a self-insured employer.

Payment Type: Refers to the method of payment of the prescription; cash, Medicaid, or third-party insurance.

PBM: Pharmacy Benefit Management Company. PBMs contract with healthcare plans to manage the pharmacy benefits of their members, from issuing pharmacy cards to full prescription adjudication.

Persistence: The adherence of the patient to the length of the drug treatment without lapses of significant length of time.

Pharmacoeconomic Studies: Research, usually sponsored by the manufacturer, to study the relationship between the cost of drugs and the clinical outcomes.

Physician Practice Management Company (PPM): A company that offers management, administrative support and capital to member physician practices for a membership fee or part of the revenue.

Plan: A drug, medical or dental benefit design.

Preferred Drug: Drug formulary status that refers to all mandatory dispensing of generics and all drugs designated as maximum allowable cost drugs.

Prevalence: The number of cases of disease, infection or other occurring at a particular point in time in relation to the population size from which it was drawn.

Primary Care Physician (PCP): A family practitioner, general internist, pediatrician, obstetrician who provides basic care and coordinates the referrals to specialists.

Prior Authorization: A process requiring a healthcare provider to obtain approval prior to providing the patient certain services and procedures. Reserved usually for services that are either expensive or likely to be overused or abused.

Prior Authorization Required Drug: Drugs that require prior approval from the plan before they are prescribed

Processor: An organization contracted with managed care plans to provide prescription benefits to enrollees.

Provider: A physician, nurse, pharmacist, hospital, group practice, nursing home, pharmacy or any individual or group of individuals that provides a healthcare service. A health plan, managed care company or insurance carrier is not a healthcare provider. Those entities are called payers. A provider may create or manage health plans, in which case, the provider is also a payer. A payer can be provider if the payer owns or manages providers, as with some staff-model HMOs.

Q-Code: temporary HCPCS level II procedure codes used for procedures, services and supplies. Q-Codes are eliminated after the assignment of permanent J-Codes.

Reimbursement: Payments received by providers or patients for benefits covered under an insurance plan.

Side effects: Problems that occur beyond the desired therapeutic effect of a treatment.

Solo Practice: A physician that practices alone without sharing of expenses and revenues with other physicians.

Step therapy: The practice of treating a medical condition with the safest and most cost-effective drug therapy and, if necessary, progressing to riskier and more costly therapies.

Third-Party Administrator (TPA): An independent organization that provides administrative services including claims processing and underwriting for other entities, such as insurance companies or employers. A TPA is either an insurance company or simply an organization with expertise and capability to administer all or a portion of the claims process.

Third Party Payer: A public or private organization that pays for health or medical expenses on behalf of beneficiaries or recipients. Beneficiaries pay a premium for such coverage in all private and in some public programs; the payer organization then pays bills on the individual's behalf. These payments are referred to as third-party payments. The three parties involved are the individual receiving the service (first party), the provider of the service (second party), and the organization paying for it (third party).

Titration: The gradual adjustment of drug dosing until the desired effect is achieved

Treatment Protocol: Specific guidelines to treat specific symptoms of a disease.

TrOOP: see True Out of Pocket Costs.

True Out of Pocket (TrOOP) Costs: Part-D patient-side costs paid by the beneficiary or on the behalf of beneficiary by an entity other than the payer.

Uniform System of Classification (USC): System for the classification of drugs designed by IMS Health.

Utilization: Use of services and supplies expressed in terms of patterns or rates of use of a single service or type of service such as hospital care, physician visits, prescription drugs, etc.

Utilization Management (UM): The evaluation of necessity, appropriateness and efficiency of healthcare services. Information is gathered on the proposed hospitalization or services from the provider and/or patient to determine whether the services meet the established guidelines and criteria.

Index

ISBN 142515900-1

9 781425 159009